# HEALTHCARE FACILITY PLANNING

T0192957

# HEALTHCARE FACILITY PLANNING

## Thinking Strategically

Cynthia Hayward

**SECOND EDITION**

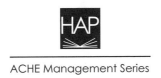

ACHE Management Series

Your board, staff, or clients may also benefit from this book's insight. For more information on quantity discounts, contact the Health Administration Press Marketing Manager at (312) 424-9450.

20   19   18   17   16         5   4   3   2   1

Library of Congress Cataloging-in-Publication Data
Names: Hayward, Cynthia, author.
Title: Healthcare facility planning : thinking strategically / Cynthia
   Hayward.
Description: Second edition. | Chicago, IL : Health Administration Press,
   [2016] | Series: ACHE management series | Includes bibliographical
   references.
Identifiers: LCCN 2016003169 (print) | LCCN 2016005884 (ebook) | ISBN
   9781567938005 (alk. paper) | ISBN 9781567938005 (E-book) | ISBN
   9781567938043 (Xml)
Subjects: LCSH: Health facilities—Design and construction. | Health
   Facilities—Planning.
Classification: LCC RA967 .H39 2016 (print) | LCC RA967 (ebook) | DDC
   725/.51—dc23
LC record available at http://lccn.loc.gov/2016003169

The paper used in this publication meets the minimum requirements of American National Standard for Information Sciences—Permanence of Paper for Printed Library Materials, ANSI Z39.48-1984. ∞ ™

Acquisitions editor: Janet Davis; Project manager: Theresa L. Rothschadl; Cover designer: Brad Norr; Layout: PerfecType

Found an error or a typo? We want to know! Please e-mail it to hapbooks@ache.org, mentioning the book's title and putting "Book Error" in the subject line.

For photocopying and copyright information, please contact Copyright Clearance Center at www.copyright .com or at (978) 750-8400.

Health Administration Press
A division of the Foundation of the American
   College of Healthcare Executives
One North Franklin Street, Suite 1700
Chicago, IL 60606-3529
(312) 424-2800

# Brief Contents

# Detailed Contents

# *Preface*

*We haven't the money, so we've got to think.*

—Lord Rutherford (1871–1937)

WHEN IT COMES to facility planning trends and capital investment, I have a tendency to divide healthcare organizations into the "haves" and the "have-nots." The haves are those well-endowed and profitable healthcare organizations that maintain a continuous cycle of renewing and regenerating their facilities. Their investments in new or renovated facilities are generally well thought out and frequently visionary, even though their capital dollars are occasionally spent on oversized or inappropriate projects. The chief executive officers and board members of these organizations often take great pride in playing the role of the master builder and point to new bricks and mortar as part of their legacy. Whether their success is the result of the genius of their strategies or is simply a function of being in the right place (market) at the right time, their customers—patients, employees, and physicians—ultimately derive substantial benefit from their expenditures.

On the other hand are the have-nots. Many healthcare organizations are still in survival mode and have not been able to focus on investing strategically in the future. In 2013, nearly one-third of community hospitals had negative operating margins and one-quarter lost money overall. Moreover, two-thirds of community hospitals lost money providing care to Medicare and Medicaid patients (American Hospital Association and Avalere Health 2014). Such financial pressures make it difficult for these healthcare organizations to make critical investments in their facilities. These organizations struggle to break even in more demographically challenged markets, experience limited negotiating leverage with payers, and find that sufficient capital is hard to obtain at their current levels of performance and cash flow. They must continue to squeeze the last bit of life out of their aging facilities with inadequate capital for retooling and renewal. Their dedicated staff use their expertise and empathy to create a healing environment. While curtailing capital spending can be a useful short-term strategy to preserve liquidity, it leads to long-term problems that are very hard to solve, including the rising age of the physical plant.

This observation is substantiated by the widening credit gap between strong and weak healthcare providers. In 2014, bond-rating downgrades for the not-for-profit healthcare sector continued to exceed upgrades. Moody's Investors Services (2015) anticipated more downgrades than upgrades in 2015.

Regardless of the financial situation, perspective, and culture of healthcare organizations, very few of them have capital to spend on inappropriate or unnecessary renovation or construction projects. Moreover, planning a major renovation project, or a new healthcare facility, is a rare opportunity for an organization to rethink its current patient care delivery model, operational systems and processes, and use of technology. A major investment of dollars in healthcare facilities should result in enhanced customer service, improved operational efficiency, potential new revenue, and increased flexibility, in addition to aesthetically pleasing, better-engineered, and code-compliant buildings that are the products of architects and engineers. At the same time, new or renovated facilities being planned today must be responsive to the needs of patients, caregivers, and payers in the twenty-first century and beyond.

The focus of this book is on predesign planning—a stage of the healthcare facility planning, design, and construction process that is frequently overlooked as organizations eagerly jump from strategic (market) planning into the more glamorous phase of design, which is typically led by an enthusiastic architect. During predesign planning, the healthcare executive has the greatest opportunity to express his or her vision for the organization, influence the nature of the process (i.e., using a top-down or a bottom-up approach), and provide input relative to the future services to be provided—their size, their location, and their financial structure. Decisions made during predesign planning also have the most impact on long-term operational costs, compared to the initial cost of the bricks and mortar. Considering that buildings constructed today may be used for a half-century or more, the time spent on predesign planning provides a disproportionately large return on investment.

The overall predesign planning process remains unchanged since the first edition of *Healthcare Facility Planning* was published in 2005. Not surprisingly, the US healthcare sector is still in a crisis. Many of the changes made in the second edition are related to the dynamic healthcare environment. Healthcare reform and new financial incentives, fluctuating utilization and demand, constant demands for technology adoption and deployment, rising turf wars among specialists, an intense focus on patient safety, and aging physical plants—all of these affect how new or renovated healthcare facilities are planned, designed, financed, and built.

This book is intended as a practical guide and is based on my 30 years' experience as a predesign planning consultant, assisting healthcare executives and boards in optimizing their facility investments and providing future flexibility. I hope that this book will help you understand the importance of the predesign planning process and tailor the process to the unique needs of your organization. By deploying an integrated facility planning process, understanding the trends that affect space allocation and configuration, and planning flexible facilities, you can move confidently from planning to implementation.

### Instructor Resources

This book's Instructor Resources include PowerPoint slides of the exhibits in the book.

For the most up-to-date information about this book and its Instructor Resources, go to ache.org/HAP and browse for the book's title or author name.

This book's Instructor Resources are available to instructors who adopt this book for use in their course. For access information, please e-mail hapbooks@ache.org.

## REFERENCES

American Hospital Association and Avalere Health. 2014. *TrendWatch Chartbook 2014: Trends Affecting Hospitals and Health Systems.* Accessed January 13, 2016. www.aha.org/research/reports/tw/chartbook/2014/14chartbook.pdf.

Moody's Investors Services. 2015. "Public Finance Upgrades Outperform in Fourth Quarter; Downgrades Prevail in 2014." Published February 10. www.moodys.com/research/Moodys-Public-finance-upgrades-outperform -in-fourth-quarter-downgrades-prevail--PR_318273.

# CHAPTER 1

# Rethinking the Facility Planning Process

WITH ALL THE dramatic changes in the healthcare industry in the past 50 years—sometimes involving 180-degree shifts in popular trends and incentives—many healthcare facilities become functionally obsolete even when their physical lives are not yet exhausted. Because of the lengthy facility planning process, new or renovated facilities that are just starting operations today may have been planned five or even ten years ago—yet these facilities are expected to endure for half a century or more. The question is, how can we ensure that the facility planning carried out this year or the next will produce facilities that are responsive to the needs of patients, caregivers, and payers in the years 2020, 2030, and beyond?

## THE TRADITIONAL FACILITY PLANNING PROCESS: PART OF THE PROBLEM

Historically, facility planning was project driven and often based on the wish lists of department managers, recruiting promises to physicians, and directives from donors. Large amounts of space and new facilities were part of the "arms race" among physicians and department managers, both internally and with competing organizations. Appreciation (or recognition in budgeting) of space as an expensive resource was limited. Capital expenditures for facilities were not always coordinated with the institution's strategic planning initiatives, operations redesign efforts, and planned information technology (IT) investments. An "if you build it, they will come" approach sometimes sufficed in lieu of a sound business plan. The impact of facility investments on long-term operational costs was frequently overlooked. Design and construction professionals tended to focus on the construction or renovation "project" and had little incentive to look for creative ways to avoid building.

1

Moreover, facility projects were seldom viewed as part of an overall capital investment strategy for the organization.

Hospitals that follow this traditional facility master planning process find that their boards deny many projects, not only because of lack of capital but also because the project's impact on operational costs is not identified. Hospital leaders must then indefinitely postpone or downsize projects, and morale suffers when they must communicate unmet expectations back to disillusioned physicians and department managers. This process often reminds me of the circus clown who opens a tin can out of which things pop out only to have to stuff the contents back into the can soon after.

When faced with a facility planning project that has taken on a life of its own, healthcare leaders must sometimes make the difficult and unpopular decision to stop or slow the planning or design process to reevaluate the need for the project and the effectiveness of the planned solution. At one critical point in the facility planning and design process, everyone involved focuses only on whether the project is "on time" and "on budget" and forgets about whether it is "on target" and is the right solution to the specific problem.

Today, successful healthcare organizations are deploying a more comprehensive, integrated, and data-driven facility planning process. This process begins with the strategic direction for the organization and integrates facility planning with market demand and service line planning, operations improvement initiatives, and anticipated investments in new technology. Major facility renovation and reconfiguration projects should be planned with a foundation of data and analyses, including business plans for key clinical service lines, a review of institution-wide operations improvement opportunities, an understanding of the project's impact on operational costs, and coordination with the organization's IT strategic plan.

## THE NEW PLANNING ENVIRONMENT

The US healthcare environment is in crisis, dealing with healthcare reform and new financial incentives, fluctuating utilization and demand, constant pressure for technology adoption and deployment, rising turf wars among specialists, an intense focus on patient safety, and aging physical plants. All of these current issues affect the way facilities are used, planned, financed, and built (Hayward 2015).

### The Impact of Healthcare Reform

The Affordable Care Act (ACA) was signed into law in 2010 with the intent of reforming the US healthcare industry. This law puts in place comprehensive health insurance reforms that roll out over several years. Some of the key provisions of this law that affect facility planning include the following:

- *Encouraging integrated healthcare.* The new law provides financial incentives for physicians to join together to form accountable care organizations (ACOs). In an ACO, physicians and various other healthcare providers take responsibility, in a collaborative and formally integrated arrangement, for coordinating the care—from prevention to acute care to chronic care and disease management—of a specific patient population.
- *Reducing paperwork and administrative costs.* Healthcare is one of the few remaining sectors that rely on paper records. The new law institutes a series of changes designed to standardize billing and requires health plans to adopt and implement rules for the secure, confidential, electronic exchange of health information. Using electronic health records (EHRs) lessens paperwork, reduces medical errors, improves the quality of care, and changes how and where many healthcare professionals do their work.
- *Bundling payments.* The law establishes a national pilot program to encourage hospitals, physicians, and other healthcare providers to work together to improve the coordination and quality of patient care. Hospitals and physicians receive a flat rate for an episode of care rather than billing each service or test separately, as in a fragmented system. The payer compensates the entire team with a "bundled" payment, which provides incentives to deliver healthcare services more efficiently while maintaining or improving quality of care.
- *Paying physicians based on value rather than volume.* A new provision ties physician payments to the quality of care they provide. Physicians see their payments modified so that those who provide higher-quality care receive higher payments than those who provide lower-quality care.
- *Improving preventive health coverage.* To expand the number of Americans receiving preventive care, the law provides new funding to state Medicaid programs that choose to cover preventive services for patients at little or no cost.

All of these changes have caused healthcare organizations to rethink the amount, type, and location of the space that is needed to deliver patient care.


## Fluctuating Demand and Utilization

Starting in the 1980s, healthcare strategists and policy experts encouraged hospitals to reduce their surplus inpatient bed capacity in response to declining admissions, use rates, and lengths of stay. These shifts had, in turn, resulted from the advent of Medicare's diagnosis-related group (or DRG) payment methodology in the public sector and managed care in the private sector. Hospitals responded to changes in demand by shifting their resources. Between 1980 and 2003, community hospitals in the United States took 175,000 inpatient beds out of service—an 18 percent reduction—through downsizing, consolidation, and closure. At the same time, skilled nursing and subacute care facilities were developed to provide a less expensive and less resource-intensive alternative for patients requiring a lengthy recuperation. Home health agencies also proliferated. After 2003, the number of hospital beds declined less dramatically. Although, nationally, inpatient admissions rose between 1992 and 2012, both the rate of inpatient admissions per 1,000 people and the average length of stay have declined to an all-time low—resulting in an overall decline in the demand for inpatient beds.

Hospitals today are at a crossroads that few had anticipated in the past. In addition to reducing the number of uninsured Americans, the ACA aims to manage a population's health across the care continuum, keeping patients healthy through preventive and primary care services and out of acute care facilities whenever possible. As healthcare transforms from a hospital-centric model to a population-centric model, and supported by sophisticated diagnostics and minimally invasive treatment, inpatient utilization may continue to decline despite the needs of aging baby boomers and the newly insured.

At the same time, ambulatory visits to community hospitals have grown dramatically over the past several decades. From 1992 to 2012, annual visits almost doubled, and the rate of growth increased as well. As the newly insured population seeks healthcare services, experts predict that ambulatory care visits will continue to grow (American Hospital Association and Avalere Health 2014), so ambulatory facilities will have to keep pace.

## The Rapid Adoption of Electronic Health Records

In the wake of new financial incentives, physician practices and hospitals may finally become paperless. The drive for EHRs in the United States started with the Health Insurance Portability and Accountability Act of 1996, which mandated the creation of a standardized method for exchanging financial and administrative healthcare information electronically. The ACA carried these initiatives even further, and the American Recovery and Reinvestment Act authorized the Centers for Medicare & Medicaid Services to provide financial incentives to encourage the adoption of EHR technology. The law required all public and private healthcare providers and other eligible professionals to have adopted and demonstrated "meaningful use" of EHRs by 2014 in order to maintain their Medicaid and Medicare reimbursement levels.

*Enterprise imaging*—in which all imaging data from disparate systems throughout the hospital are available in one place via the patient's EHR—is likely the next development in EHR storage and management. This shift will take the responsibility for imaging management from radiology and make it an enterprisewide IT function. With this evolution, all clinical data are available, easily accessible, and usable, allowing organizations to provide coordinated patient care that is not confined to department silos.

## Advances in Information Technology

The healthcare environment will increasingly rely on data, whether in the form of EHRs, financial and management information, imaging studies, sensor and device readings, voice communications, or telemedicine. Continued advances in IT are creating new staff positions and job descriptions and altering historical perceptions regarding necessary functional relationships. Hospital leaders are consolidating traditional health and financial data management functions (e.g., medical records, quality assurance, risk management, infection control, finance, data processing, telecommunications) as data become increasingly computerized and common databases generate data more quickly and effectively. At the same time, new interdisciplinary fields are evolving—such as health informatics—that will require healthcare professionals to have the skills and knowledge necessary to develop, implement, and manage IT software and applications in a medical environment.

The creation of a paperless healthcare environment that exploits Internet, mobile, and wireless technologies is having a revolutionary impact on the need for physical proximity between departments and functional areas. Many of the traditional facility planning principles that were based on the need for departments to share paper, equipment, and patients are no longer relevant.

## The Convergence of Diagnostic and Interventional Imaging and Surgical Procedures

While imaging procedures are becoming more interventional and no longer limited to diagnostic procedures, surgery is becoming less invasive. For many years, real-time imaging, using a mobile ultrasound or endoscopy unit (also called a *C-arm*, a name derived from its shape), has been a standard part of the surgical operating room. Today, the hybrid operating room has permanently installed equipment such as intraoperative computed tomography (CT), magnetic resonance imaging (MRI), and fixed C-arms. Physicians typically use these machines in conjunction with cardiovascular, thoracic, neurosurgery, spinal, and orthopedic procedures to enable diagnostic imaging before, during, and after a surgical procedure. This insight allows the surgeon to assess the effectiveness of the surgery and perform further resections or additional interventions in a single encounter. Many equipment vendors now offer highly specialized, proprietary imaging systems that are integrated with the operating room, while others offer designs that position the CT or MRI with dual access so that the equipment can be used independently for diagnostic procedures when surgery is not in progress.

## Turf Wars

Interventional radiologists—using their expertise in angioplasty and catheter-delivered stents to treat peripheral arterial disease—were the first minimally invasive specialists. As cardiologists and vascular surgeons increased their use of interventional techniques, territorial disputes emerged. The specialties of interventional radiology, interventional cardiology, and endovascular surgical neuroradiology are all perfecting the use of stents and other procedures to keep diseased arteries open, and they are evaluating new applications. The rapid development of new imaging technologies, mechanical devices, and different treatment options, while certainly beneficial to the patient, can also lead to ambiguity regarding specific specialty claims on certain techniques and devices. These practitioners are often in competition with each other, creating "turf" wars. As a consequence, workloads—and the need for space—may fluctuate depending on how, by whom, and where a specific procedure is performed.

## The Reengineering of Operations and Ongoing Process Improvement

With continued pressures to reduce the cost of labor as well as other expensive resources, healthcare organizations are expanding manager and supervisor responsibilities and merging departments to share staff, equipment, and space. Human resources departments are revising narrowly defined job descriptions to reflect opportunities for cross-training and increased responsibilities. The resulting new organizational charts are becoming compressed and flatter.

Improving patient throughput allows healthcare organizations to optimize their resources, often using Lean process improvement. Lean is a customer-centric methodology used to continually improve any process through the elimination of waste. The approach involves establishing a baseline by defining the current state of operations and then using industry trends, best practices, benchmarks, and other metrics to define the desired future state. When applied to facility planning, an organization typically focuses first on improving operations, apart from making any physical improvements. Once Lean processes are established, planners can begin looking at how physical improvements might further enable operational improvements. An iterative approach is necessary to reaching consensus on the appropriate balance between improving operational processes and investing capital in facilities.

## Consolidation

The US healthcare delivery system has been undergoing consolidation for many years. Healthcare reform may propel this trend by providing financial incentives for developing ACOs and implementing EHRs and by encouraging providers to share risk with bundled payments. In 2013, the number of hospitals and hospital beds involved in mergers reached a five-year high (American Hospital Association and Avalere Health 2014). In addition, healthcare systems are acquiring physician practices, outpatient surgery centers, and imaging centers at a record pace. The remaining independent physicians are joining forces and assembling into large, multispecialty group practices. Radiology "supergroups" are also evolving to compete locally, as well as nationally, which is made possible by teleradiology technology that allows 24/7 instant access to images from any location. Healthcare systems are also reorganizing physically and operationally by specific diseases or service lines—frequently with a center-of-excellence orientation—to optimize capital investments in expensive technologies, attract leading-edge physicians, and better market their services.

## Reimbursement's Impact on Service Demand and Location

Since 2008, the healthcare environment has experienced a reverse migration of sorts. Healthcare organizations are increasingly acquiring private physician offices and ambulatory surgery and diagnostic centers and converting them to hospital outpatient departments. The goal is to optimize reimbursement for hospitals, lessen the risk for their owners, and, ideally, improve the coordination of patient care.

## Intense Media Attention to Patient Safety

In December 1999, the Institute of Medicine (IOM 2000), an arm of the National Academy of Sciences, published *To Err Is Human*, a report that estimates that some

98,000 deaths and more than a million injuries occur each year as a result of medical errors. Following the publication of this IOM report, additional studies at major medical universities and healthcare organizations around the world have advanced our understanding of how these medical errors occur. Medical professionals widely believe that the original estimates were significantly understated simply because the data were not captured or reported effectively in most organizations. The focus on patient safety has led healthcare organizations to redesign work processes, implement new technologies, and rethink the design and layout of key spaces. The rapid adoption of bar coding, the emphasis on medication safety zones, and the use of standardized layouts for inpatient rooms and treatment spaces are all a result of patient-safety concerns.

## Aging Facilities

Healthcare organizations, like most businesses, need to continually maintain and update their physical plants, upgrade and retool their facilities to meet changing demand, and invest in new technologies. However, the investment required for healthcare facilities today is staggering because of the high costs of technology deployment, regulatory compliance, and upgrading physical plants for which ongoing maintenance may have been deferred for decades. Hospital facilities are aging: In 2010, the average age of the plant was about 10 years. By 2014, the average age increased to almost 11 years, which indicates that there is insufficient investment in healthcare facilities (Garber 2014).

## The New Consumerism

At the same time that the healthcare industry is experiencing intense pressures to reduce costs, limited access to capital for facility upgrading or replacement, and capacity issues with an expanding population of the newly insured, a new consumer-driven market is emerging, fueled in part by aging baby boomers. Better educated than their parents and empowered by the Internet, baby boomers not only have the analytical ability to review research and form an opinion about treatment options, but they may also spend substantial discretionary income on their healthcare needs.

At the same time, younger consumers are paying a greater proportion of their healthcare insurance premiums and medical bills as employers shift more costs to employees. The shift by large employers from a defined benefit to a defined contribution is resulting in a consumer-led market that encourages consumers to become prudent purchasers of healthcare insurance and medical services.

## UNDERSTANDING THE NEW VOCABULARY

Rethinking the facility planning process also requires the use of new terminology, as shown in exhibit 1.1. Strategic planning has become more focused on financial viability, so healthcare organizations should rely on a *capital investment strategy* rather than the traditional facility master plan to balance the trade-offs between investments in new bricks-and-mortar buildings, medical equipment and IT, ventures with physicians, and so on. Space planning, particularly for a major clinical service line, cannot be accomplished without *operations improvement, technology investment*, and a *business (market) plan* that describes the market dynamics. I prefer to use the term *operational and space programming* to describe the traditional space planning process, instead of the more common term *functional and space programming*, to emphasize the rigor that is required in rethinking operational processes before planning the physical space.

Even the traditional equipment planning process has changed. Most major equipment items use digital technology that must dovetail with the organization's

---

**Exhibit 1.1 Understanding the New Facility Planning Vocabulary**

| Old | | New |
|-----|---|-----|
| Facility master plan | ➡ | Capital investment strategy |
| Space planning | ➡ | Business/market planning<br>Operations improvement<br>Technology investment |
| | | ⬇ |
| | | Operational (functional)<br>and space programming |
| Equipment planning | ➡ | Equipment/technology planning |
| Bricks and mortar | ➡ | Physical and virtual spaces |

---

*Source:* Reprinted from Hayward (2015).

overall information management and technology strategy. With electronic information exchange replacing the traditional flow of paper (and people), facility planners are reevaluating physical proximities that were once considered necessary and identifying new settings for delivering patient care. As a result, the traditional bricks-and-mortar concept is being replaced by a combination of *physical and virtual spaces*.

## THE CHALLENGE OF PREDESIGN PLANNING

The planning and delivery of a major capital project can be divided into six stages, as shown in exhibit 1.2. The first stage of predesign planning—the focus of this book—includes general concepts and ideas in the form of words, numbers, and conceptual diagrams. Planners use preliminary space estimates to develop a facility master plan and generate project cost estimates early. Once specific projects are identified and approved, the detailed operational and space programming begins;

**Exhibit 1.2 Six Stages of a Capital Project**

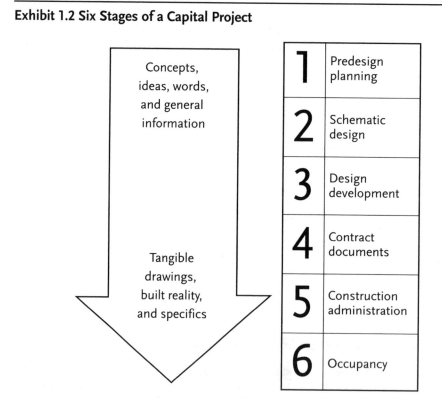

*Source:* Reprinted with permission from Waite, P. S. 2005. *The Non-Architect's Guide to Major Capital Projects: Planning, Designing, and Delivering New Buildings.* Ann Arbor, MI: Society for College and University Planning.

when this process is completed, the design architect can start the schematic design stage. Each subsequent phase brings more knowledge and detail about the project and has its own cast of players. Nearing the final phases, the concepts and ideas are translated into tangible architectural floor plans, drawings of construction details, and the eventual reality of the three-dimensional building (Waite 2005).

Predesign planning is the process of determining the following (Hayward 2015):

- The *right services* consistent with the organization's strategic initiatives, market dynamics, and business plan, at the
- *right size* based on projected demand, staffing, equipment, technology, and desired amenities, in the
- *right location* based on access, operational efficiency, and building suitability, with the
- *right financial structure* (e.g., owning, leasing, or partnering).

Predesign planning is the stage at which the healthcare executive has the most influence on the potential success of the final project. Her opportunity for input decreases as each subsequent stage passes. The opportunity to reduce both the initial capital cost and the ongoing operational costs is also greatest during the predesign planning stage, as shown in exhibit 1.3. With the prospect of a new building project, healthcare executives tend to short-circuit or bypass the predesign stage to rush into the more tangible aspect of design. This is a big mistake. A premature focus on a construction or renovation project, without the rigor of the predesign planning process and the context of an overall capital investment strategy for the organization, often results in inappropriate and overbuilt facilities and increased operational costs that may not be justified by revenue growth. This move is also a mistake, given that you, your organization, and your predecessors will have to live with the results of your project for a half-century or more. Predesign planning is critical from a short-term perspective: It is needed to design and construct a building that meets the needs of the first set of occupants. Predesign planning is also critical to the building's long-range functional life and its adaptability to future changes in medical practice, technology, and patient care.

According to Phillip S. Waite (2005, 1–2), predesign planning is the part of the process during which nonarchitects are the most involved. He cautions against engaging a design consultant prematurely: "Architects and engineers are energetic, creative problem solvers who are really good at what they do. But until your institution has worked through some of the steps of predesign, you don't know if your problem is really a design problem or some other kind of problem. There are architects who tend to see all problems as design problems, even when they are actually management or organizational problems. A management or organization problem

**Exhibit 1.3 Impact of Predesign Planning on Potential Capital and Operational Costs**

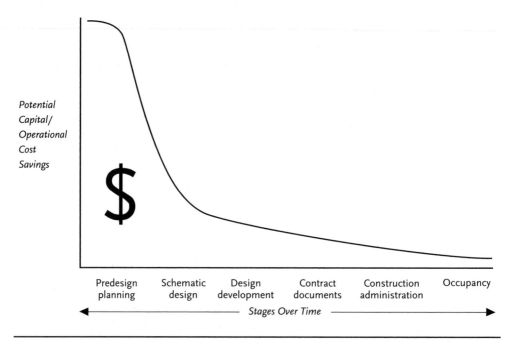

can often be solved internally by a policy decision rather than a design, thus saving a lot of time and money."

## THE INTEGRATED PREDESIGN PLANNING PROCESS

Exhibit 1.4 illustrates the integrated predesign planning process that can be used by healthcare organizations to reconfigure existing facilities and to plan new facilities. The predesign planning activities shown in the diagram are separated into two phases that are explained in the next sections:

1. *Capital investment strategy development and approval* include six major activities (replacing the traditional facility master planning process).
2. *Implementation* includes the detailed operational and space programming for designated projects and the establishment of benchmarks to monitor long-range facility needs as the strategy is periodically updated.

**Exhibit 1.4 The Integrated Predesign Planning Process**

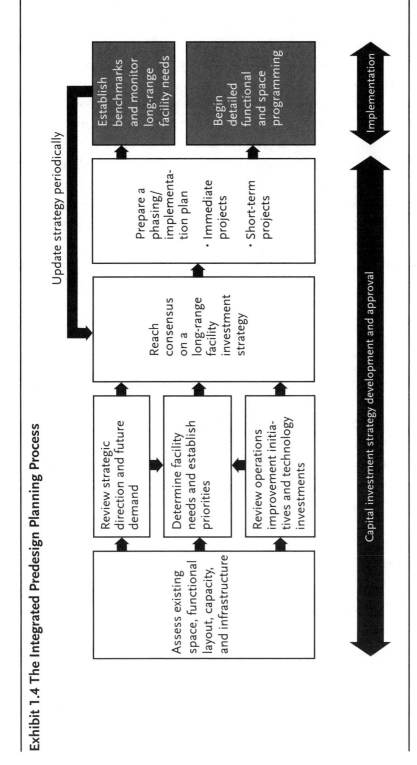

*Source:* Reprinted from Hayward (2015).

### Capital Investment Strategy Development and Approval

The predesign process begins with the collection of baseline facility data and a review of the organization's current situation, including campus access and circulation, bed use and configuration, space allocation and layout, and infrastructure issues. Current market dynamics, workload trends, future vision, and projected demand should also be reviewed and incorporated into the facility planning process, along with the organization's institution-wide and service line–specific operations improvement initiatives. Planned technology investments should be concurrently reviewed and coordinated with the facility planning process.

Existing and future space needs should be documented and compared with current space allocation. At this point, future facility needs must be determined, priorities must be established, and consensus must be reached on a long-range facility investment strategy. Once the long-range facility investment strategy, or "road map," is defined, it can be divided or categorized into immediate, short-term, and long-range projects, which are assigned corresponding capital requirements that are sequenced over a multiyear period.

### Implementation

With the phasing and implementation plan in hand, detailed operational (functional) and space programming can begin for those projects that are identified as immediate priorities, along with short-term projects for which planning needs to begin so that they can be completed within a two- to five-year planning horizon. Benchmarks are established for long-range projects; these benchmarks can be monitored over time and incorporated into the ongoing predesign planning process as the facility investment strategy is updated periodically.

## THE PREDESIGN PLANNING TEAM

The hospital leadership needs to assemble a facility planning committee or task force, which is typically led by the chief executive officer, chief operating officer, or another designated senior executive in the organization. An outside consultant who has unique expertise in predesign planning may also lead the group. At the predesign planning stage, the facility planning committee generally includes the members of the existing management team and representatives from the medical staff and the building committee of the board. In addition, the organization's facility manager should be part of the team. The committee structure will ultimately reflect the organization's culture (top-down approach or bottom-up approach) but should not become overly large. A group of 9–12 members is manageable and provides a sufficient diversity of representation. The team will generally meet on a monthly basis but may meet more often, depending on the unique issues at hand.

Bringing a design architect or construction manager on board at the onset of the predesign planning stage is not necessary. Using an architect or facility planning consultant who is focused exclusively on predesign planning is desirable and prevents the potential conflict of interest associated with having the predesign planning process led by the firm that will ultimately be charged with the design or construction (and compensated at a percentage of the project cost). This precaution is particularly relevant during the detailed operational and space programming phase.

If the organization has an *architect of record* (who often resides in the community, has had a long-term relationship with the organization, and has extensive knowledge of the physical plant), the committee should consider her a valuable member of the predesign planning team.

Establishing the role of the committee is vital. The facility planning committee is typically responsible for prequalifying and selecting external consultants, reviewing and validating baseline data, confirming and challenging perceptions regarding facility deficiencies, and validating institution-wide and service line–specific operational assumptions. The committee will also be responsible for translating the organization's vision into facility needs and priorities as well as for shaping the organization's long-range facility investment strategy. Once the committee reaches consensus on this strategy, it should communicate the decision to the rest of the organization. In particular, the designated nursing and medical staff representatives must be able to educate their respective constituencies and act as emissaries to communicate and promote the benefits of the plan.

In some cases, healthcare organizations may need specific feasibility studies as part of the predesign planning stage and may require additional consultants, depending on in-house resources. These studies may include a determination of whether a proposed project is financially, legally, or physically feasible. The facility planning committee may ask an architectural design consultant or construction specialist to perform specific feasibility studies when a new or replacement healthcare facility is planned—for example, a site analysis—or when extensive facility renewal or replacement is required on a constrained site, and multiple architectural and engineering solutions may need to be evaluated. Such use of a design architect during the predesign planning process should not be confused with the subsequent stage of schematic design. Planners should make clear to the selected design, engineering, or construction consultants that their work during the predesign planning stage is not a guarantee of future involvement in the subsequent design and construction of the proposed building project.

The facility planning committee is usually charged with prequalifying and selecting the design architect, construction manager, and other specialty consultants at the end of the predesign planning stage.

Once all predesign planning activities have been accomplished and the organization is ready to start the next stage—schematic design—the following books may be consulted as references:

- *The Non-Architect's Guide to Major Capital Projects: Planning, Designing, and Delivering New Buildings* by Phillip S. Waite (2005). This book addresses the design and construction process, contracting approaches, and the project delivery team.
- *Launching a Capital Facility Project: A Guide for Healthcare Leaders* by John E. Kemper (2010). This book is a good resource when an organization is planning a new or replacement hospital project.

## REFERENCES

American Hospital Association and Avalere Health. 2014. *TrendWatch Chartbook 2014: Trends Affecting Hospitals and Health Systems*. Accessed January 13, 2016. www.aha.org/research/reports/tw/chartbook/2014/14chartbook.pdf.

Garber, K. M. 2014. "Average Age of Plant: Hospitals About 11 Years." *American Hospital Association Resource Center Blog*. Originally posted October 20, 2011. https://aharesourcecenter.wordpress.com/tag/average-age-of-plant/.

Hayward, C. 2015. *SpaceMed Guide: A Space Planning Guide for Healthcare Facilities*, 3rd ed. Ann Arbor, MI: HA Ventures.

Institute of Medicine (IOM). 2000. *To Err Is Human: Building a Safer Health System*. Washington, DC: National Academies Press.

Kemper, J. E. 2010. *Launching a Capital Facility Project: A Guide for Healthcare Leaders*, 2nd ed. Chicago: Health Administration Press.

Waite, P. S. 2005. *The Non-Architect's Guide to Major Capital Projects: Planning, Designing, and Delivering New Buildings*. Ann Arbor, MI: Society for College and University Planning.

# CHAPTER 2

# Understanding Your Current Facility

COLLECTING AND ANALYZING data on your current facility is the first step in preparing a long-range capital investment strategy. Knowing your facility's current site access and circulation, layout and configuration, space allocation, and physical condition will allow you to identify key issues and establish priorities. Assessing the success of a major renovation or construction project is very difficult without a thorough understanding of the baseline conditions.

Key questions to ask when analyzing the facility may include the following:

- How much land do we occupy, and how do our customers access our site and facilities?
- What type of space do we have, and where is it located?
- How many beds do we have, and how are they organized?
- How many and what types of diagnostic and treatment spaces do we use? How much space are we currently using?
- What ongoing investment will we require for infrastructure upgrading and future maintenance of our physical plant?

## WORKING FROM THE OUTSIDE INWARD

Evaluating the current facility should begin with a review of overall property boundaries and site access points. Designated campus circulation routes and corresponding parking areas should be identified by type of traffic, such as emergency vehicles, service trucks, patients, and visitors. The number of parking spaces available by type (if restricted) should also be tabulated. In addition, potential areas for physical expansion and expansion constraints—such as underground utilities, easements, and covenants—should be identified. Key building entrances should also be noted.

Every healthcare campus must accommodate the flow of a variety of customers, including patients, visitors, staff, and physicians; ambulance and emergency traffic; and service traffic. Identifying and tracking the different types of circulation facilitates a wayfinding assessment. *Wayfinding* begins with the customer's arrival on the campus, and it involves signage and visual cues to assist customers in identifying the appropriate building entrance, finding parking if necessary, and arriving at the desired service location.

Expediting campus access for emergency vehicles and emergency patients arriving by private vehicle is particularly important in designing a campus that facilitates wayfinding. Signage may direct outpatients to a medical office building, a hospital-based clinic, or a diagnostic area for a routine visit or procedure and may also direct outpatients to a surgery or special procedure center, after which they may require an extended recovery or admission. Most healthcare campuses also accommodate outpatients with chronic conditions who require recurring care, such as physical therapy or dialysis, and may need to navigate the hospital campus frequently. Unless admitted through the emergency department (ED), most patients today arrive at the hospital as outpatients and are generally admitted postprocedure.

In addition to patient traffic, the healthcare campus must accommodate visitors and family members who may arrive separately or who may drop off a patient, park, and then reunite. A well-designed circulation system must be provided for hospital employees and physicians who need to park and access their workplaces. The site should include a separate circulation system for service traffic, such as delivery trucks and trash pickup, to access the loading dock. Service traffic should not be visible to patients and visitors and should certainly not impede ambulance and emergency traffic.

## ALL SPACE IS NOT THE SAME

An early understanding of the different types of space within a healthcare facility, their general characteristics, the factors influencing space need, and current space planning trends (summarized in exhibit 2.1) is necessary. Different types, or categories, of space may have varying building code compliance requirements, renovation or construction costs, and reuse potential.

### Inpatient Nursing Units

Based on my experience, these units generally occupy 35–40 percent of the total usable space in a community hospital. This type of space must comply with the most stringent hospital building codes for egress during a fire or other disaster because it is occupied by extended length of stay patients who are not ambulatory. In an era

**Exhibit 2.1 Characteristics of Different Types of Space in a Healthcare Facility**

| Category of Space | Facility Characteristics | Space Drivers | Current Trends |
|---|---|---|---|
| Inpatient nursing units | • Modular construction<br>• Limited flexibility for cost-effective reuse<br>• Most stringent code requirements due to patient acuity and extended length of stay<br>• Revenue generating | • Patient-care delivery model<br>• Acuity and length of stay<br>• Unit size<br>• Type of patient accommodations<br>• Technology and operational systems<br>• Facility layout and design<br>• Desired amenities | • Increasing patient acuity<br>• Transition to electronic communications and increased automation<br>• Flexible design for alternate levels of care<br>• Facility layout designed to optimize scarce nursing personnel<br>• Demand for private rooms |
| Diagnostic and treatment space | • Generally accommodates inpatients and outpatients unless outpatient volume justifies redundant equipment, staff, space<br>• More stringent code requirements with inpatient occupancy<br>• Some modalities are expensive to build and have unique architectural design requirements (e.g., operating rooms, interventional imaging, magnetic resonance imaging); other modalities use miniaturized, mobile equipment<br>• Rapidly changing technology<br>• Revenue generating | • Organization structure<br>• Patient mix<br>• Technology and operational concepts<br>• Throughput of equipment<br>• Average versus peak workloads<br>• Scheduling patterns<br>• Number of physician and administrative offices<br>• Recruitment promises | • Rapid advances in technology and melding or blurring of modalities<br>• Extended hours of operation to optimize equipment utilization<br>• Optimizing flexibility and sharing of resources (e.g., equipment, staff, space)<br>• Shift to point-of-care services with miniaturized, more mobile equipment<br>• Networking with physician offices<br>• Advances in telemedicine (e.g., patient remote from specialty physician or technician)<br>• Increased "stat" and 24/7 requests to facilitate throughput and shorten length of stay |
| Customer service space and amenities | • First point of entry or contact for patients and their families<br>• Typically includes a variety of "departments" and amenities (e.g., lobbies or lounges)<br>• Cost of space varies with amenities desired | • Institutional policy<br>• Department/organization structure<br>• Overall traffic volume and circulation or flow patterns<br>• Scope of retail activities | • Replication of "hotel" reception desk (hub and spoke) model<br>• Focus on first impression or image<br>• Operational restructuring around needs of customer |

**Exhibit 2.1 Characteristics of Different Types of Space in a Healthcare Facility (Continued)**

| Category of Space | Facility Characteristics | Space Drivers | Current Trends |
|---|---|---|---|
| Clinical support space | • Minimal patient traffic<br>• Specialized design considerations<br>• Increased use of robotics (e.g., laboratory, pharmacy)<br>• Shift of services to point of care | • Equipment and technology more critical than workload volume<br>• Staffing on the primary shift | • Increased automation and use of robotics, bar coding, and so on<br>• Unbundling services to less expensive space |
| Physician practice space | • Ambulatory patient traffic<br>• Less expensive construction<br>• Significant parking requirements<br>• Demand depends on who pays for space | • Scope of diagnostic procedures and treatments<br>• Workload and scheduling patterns<br>• Shared versus exclusive-use space<br>• Number and location of physician administrative offices | • Time-share space, with more efficient scheduling of exam and treatment space<br>• Extended hours of operation<br>• Competition for outpatients, with convenient access and contiguous parking<br>• Variable impact of reimbursement on service locations and facility configuration |
| Administrative office space | • Typically generic office space; not revenue producing<br>• Limited patient and visitor traffic<br>• Least stringent code requirements<br>• Less costly to build or renovate | • Organization structure<br>• Staff on primary (day) shift<br>• Shared versus exclusive-use space | • Reorganization of traditional departments to optimize sharing of resources<br>• Creation of generic office space and consolidation in less-expensive space |
| Building support space | • No patient traffic<br>• Generally open, industrial space<br>• Least costly construction (except kitchen)<br>• Inpatient units are primary users<br>• Services should be opaque to customers | • Primarily hospital beds<br>• Organizational structure and operational concepts<br>• Equipment and technology<br>• Make, buy, sell decisions | • Shift to point-of-care and on-demand services<br>• Unbundling of services into less expensive space (e.g., service building)<br>• Advances in technology (e.g., robotics, bar coding, radio-frequency identification)<br>• Outsourcing |

of fluctuating demand, high labor costs, evolving technology, and limited access to capital, the management of this large amount of space is a significant issue for most healthcare organizations. Inpatient nursing units represent a major portion of an organization's revenue base (and operational costs), and the construction or renovation of inpatient nursing units is expensive compared with that of other types of space.

The layout of a typical inpatient floor is based on a common patient room module, which includes a fixed plumbing chase to support a contiguous patient bathroom. Building codes require all patient rooms to have windows to admit natural light. Staff and visitors access patient rooms from a horizontal circulation corridor (eight feet wide at a minimum) that leads to elevator lobbies and stairwells that, in turn, provide vertical circulation to the rest of the facility. Patient rooms are supplemented by various support spaces (which do not require natural light) that are placed in an inner-core area.

Patient acuity and length of stay are the primary factors that affect the number of beds, the size of the patient room, and the corresponding support space. Higher-acuity patients or extended-stay patients require additional space. Larger patient rooms are required for sicker patients who may require emergency intervention or treatments that involve additional equipment and staff. Although they do not require larger patient rooms, inpatient units for extended lengths of stay—for example, psychiatric units and skilled nursing units—must provide additional support space for group dining, therapy, and family visitation, according to current guidelines (Facilities Guidelines Institute 2014).

The size of a specific nursing unit, which is defined as a group of patient rooms that shares a central nursing station and support space (along with a single nurse manager and unit clerk), is also influenced by the mix of private and semiprivate patient rooms, planned operational and technical support systems, and the level of amenities desired. However, the optimal number of beds on a given nursing unit or floor is related to the modular divisibility of the total number of beds. For example, a 32-bed nursing unit can be divided into subunits of 4, 6, or 8 beds, or it can be divided into 2 subunits of 16 beds. Facility planners are developing flexible designs that can accommodate alternate staffing patterns and levels of care either by shift or over time to minimize future renovation if the patient population changes.

Because of the modular nature of an inpatient unit, this type of space poses a challenge when healthcare organizations consider conversion to noninpatient use. Reassignment for an alternate functional use either results in an inefficient use of space (when the space is reused without physical reconfiguration) or involves high renovation costs (when walls and utility chases are moved). Because the rigid column and bay spacing and numerous fixed utility chases often make major reconfiguration cost prohibitive, most organizations find that they are limited to infrastructure upgrades and cosmetic renovations of nursing units.

When inpatient space is either no longer needed or has become functionally obsolete, a common practice is to redeploy or downgrade the space for administrative offices. However, compared with building or leasing space in an office building, this practice requires more space to house a given number of offices because of wider corridors, fixed columns, and the proliferation of toilet and bathing facilities—all of which are expensive to renovate. Higher operational costs also result, because the surplus space still must be cleaned, maintained, insured, and secured.

## Diagnostic and Treatment Space

This space typically accommodates inpatients and outpatients. When outpatient workload volumes are sufficient to justify redundant resources—equipment, staff, and space—or when necessitated by market dynamics and strategic partnering, healthcare organizations may develop dedicated or freestanding outpatient facilities. Procedure rooms may need to be designed for sophisticated digital equipment with unique design and environmental requirements—for example, lead shielding or reinforced floors—or they may require no more than an exam table, sink, and storage cabinetry to support a small piece of portable equipment.

As with inpatient nursing units, diagnostic and treatment services are a source of revenue and are therefore frequent targets of expansion when healthcare organizations anticipate incremental demand. In addition to current and projected workloads, the patient mix, level of technology, operational concepts, throughput of the equipment, scheduling patterns, and overall organizational structure all affect the amount of space needed. The fulfillment of recruitment promises to physicians also frequently drives the type of equipment and amount of space allocated.

Because of rapid advances in new technology, minimally invasive diagnostic and treatment capabilities, the shift to point-of-care services, and the blending and melding of some of the traditional imaging modalities, healthcare organizations are increasingly focusing on long-range flexibility when constructing diagnostic and treatment space. The trend is toward creation of generic "large" and "small" procedure rooms that can accommodate varying equipment over time and are supported by shared patient intake, preparation, and recovery areas.

## Customer Services and Amenities

Such space is used by multiple departments and staff involved in assisting the patient, family members, and others with navigating the array of healthcare services both on- and off-site. Space in this category generally includes areas for reception, admitting and registration, central scheduling, cashiering, insurance verification, physician referrals, and various similar services. This category of space also includes amenities such as lobbies, lounges, gift shops, cafés, and libraries or resource centers that may be found in any hospitality facility (a hotel, for example). Unfortunately, many acute care hospitals still organize these services according to their traditional departments rather than around the needs of the patients and other customers. Many of these departments are located on the first floor of the healthcare facility (which is prime real estate), even though only a small number of staff actually have face-to-face contact with patients and their families.

Space need is influenced primarily by the organization of these services and the number of staff who require workstations. Institutional policies regarding the amount and scope of amenities provided and the intended ambiance also affect the space allocation in any given facility. Key trends include replicating the hotel reception–desk concept (hub-and-spoke model) to enhance customer satisfaction and creating a positive first impression on initial entry into the facility. Support space for other customers may include staff lockers and lounges, fitness facilities, and day care centers for employees' children.

## Clinical Support Space

This space includes the clinical laboratory, pharmacy, central sterile processing, and similar services that, although unique to a healthcare facility, do not accommodate patient traffic as diagnostic and treatment services do. Space need, physical con-figuration, and location are determined primarily by the type of equipment and technology deployed rather than by actual workload. Significant developments in automation and robotics, bar coding, and information management have drastically altered the way this type of space is planned today. With efficient delivery systems in place for specimens, medications, and instruments, to name a few, many of these clinical support services are being relocated to less expensive, industrial-style space.

## Physician Practice Space

This space typically consists of a patient reception (intake) area; a large number of identical exam rooms; a small number of offices, consultation rooms, and special procedure rooms; and accompanying support space. Construction of physician practice space, which is exclusively used by outpatients who are ambulatory, is less expensive than the other types of patient care space described earlier. Physician practice space may be located in a medical office building (either freestanding or connected to an acute care hospital); colocated with diagnostic and treatment services in a comprehensive ambulatory care center; or become part of an institute or center of excellence organized along a specific service line such as cardiology, cancer, orthopedics, or geriatrics.

Physicians may own their office space, lease dedicated space, participate in a time-share arrangement, or work in hospital-sponsored clinics. The size and configuration of the space vary, depending on the medical practice model and scheduling patterns, the workload volumes and exam room turnaround, and the scope of diagnostic and treatment procedures.

Physician practice space is often located in one or more freestanding buildings on a healthcare campus (typical of specialists) to provide contiguous patient parking and convenient access or distributed throughout the community (which is typical of primary care physicians). Because most physicians use relatively generic space, time-share concepts are becoming increasingly popular as a way to optimize use of space and minimize the rental and operational costs borne by the individual physician or group practice.

## Administrative Offices

This space is used by many hospital departments involved in the administration and management of the organization. Regardless of the department assignment, this space generally includes a mix of private offices, enclosed or semi-enclosed cubicles, and open workstations to accommodate different hierarchies of staff as dictated by the organizational structure. Patient and family traffic is rare in such spaces. Employees occupy much of the administrative space only during standard business hours, and the number of staff and the organizational structure dictate the amount of space required. Operational reengineering and advancements in information technology in the past decade have reduced the number of administrative staff. At the same time, every new program requires some amount of office space, and the consolidation of existing services often results in the need for a larger block of space in a single location.

## Building Support

This space is required for those services that support any large industrial or hospitality complex, and it includes materials management, environmental services, and food services. Space for these services should function efficiently in the background and be invisible to patients and visitors. These services use open, industrial-style space that, with the exception of the kitchen, is perhaps the least costly space to construct and renovate, assuming that it is not integrated with the hospital chassis in such a way that it must be built or maintained to more stringent hospital codes. Kitchen space, on the other hand, is among the most expensive space per square foot to construct on the healthcare campus.

The need for building support space is primarily driven by the number of inpatients; the equipment and technology to be deployed; and the decisions by the organization to make, buy, or sell these services. The unbundling of these services into inexpensive, industrial-style space and the increased use of automated distribution systems, robotics, and electronic materials management and inventory systems also affect the size and configuration of the space.

## Other Space

"Other" categories may include research and education spaces. Such spaces are an integral part of most academic medical centers but not commonly found in community hospitals, with the exception of space for clinical trials and centralized or decentralized conference and training facilities. The need for research space is driven by program funding and recruiting promises. The required amount of education space depends on the healthcare organization's specific educational programs, scheduling patterns, and typical number of participants. In-service education on the healthcare campus is being redefined with the increased use of distance-learning concepts such as videoconferencing, Internet meetings and presentations, and self-directed learning. At the same time, the proliferation of sophisticated medical technologies is creating new demands for in-service education. Some healthcare organizations, however, opt to lease space (as needed) at local community centers, hotels, or schools in lieu of constructing large meeting rooms or an auditorium for infrequent use.

## DIFFERENTIATING BETWEEN NET SPACE AND GROSS SPACE

Frequent misunderstandings arise when hospital leaders, department staff, planners, and architects confuse *net square feet* with *gross square feet*. As shown in exhibit 2.2, net square feet (NSF) refers to the inside, wall-to-wall dimensions within a room or area and represents the actual usable space. The total of the NSF of all usable rooms and areas in a department is referred to as the *department net square feet* (DNSF). However, the most common term used in facility master planning is

# Exhibit 2.2 Comparison of Net Square Feet and Gross Square Feet

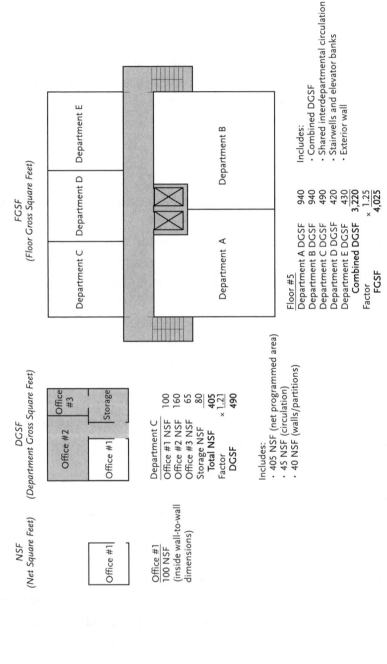

NSF
*(Net Square Feet)*

DGSF
*(Department Gross Square Feet)*

FGSF
*(Floor Gross Square Feet)*

Office #1

Office #1
100 NSF
(inside wall-to-wall dimensions)

Department C
Office #1 NSF    100
Office #2 NSF    160
Office #3 NSF     65
Storage NSF       80
**Total NSF**    **405**
Factor         × 1.21
**DGSF**         **490**

Includes:
· 405 NSF (net programmed area)
· 45 NSF (circulation)
· 40 NSF (walls/partitions)

Floor #5
Department A DGSF    940
Department B DGSF    940
Department C DGSF    490
Department D DGSF    420
Department E DGSF    430
**Combined DGSF**  **3,220**
Factor             × 1.25
**FGSF**           **4,025**

Includes:
· Combined DGSF
· Shared interdepartmental circulation
· Stairwells and elevator banks
· Exterior wall

*Source:* Reprinted from Hayward (2015).

*department gross square feet* (DGSF), which represents the "footprint" of the specific department. DGSF includes the space occupied by internal circulation corridors, walls and partitions, and minor utility columns, in addition to the usable NSF in the department. DGSF excludes common areas such as shared public corridors and lobbies, elevator banks, stairwells, major mechanical spaces, the space occupied by the building's exterior wall, central toilet facilities, housekeeping, equipment storage, and other shared space.

To convert the sum of all net spaces to an estimate of the actual department footprint, a *net-to-department gross space conversion factor* is used. The estimated DGSF is used to test the feasibility of different facility configuration options during facility master planning and to estimate renovation costs prior to design.

Net-to-department gross space conversion factors generally range from 1.20 to 1.50. Large, open spaces—for example, those usually planned for building support services such as materials management and environmental services—would have a lower factor because of a limited number of walls and partitions and minimal internal corridors. A surgery suite would have a larger factor to account for numerous and variously sized rooms that must be connected by eight-foot-wide corridors to accommodate patients' stretchers. The factor for a specific functional area will also vary depending on whether new construction is planned (lower factor) or if the function is to be retrofitted into existing space with specific design constraints (higher factor). Constraints—such as the shape of the existing building envelope, minimal bay width and unusual column spacing, and fixed mechanical spaces and pipe shafts—may require a greater amount of DGSF to accommodate the same amount of NSF than in new construction.

Additional factors are used to estimate the overall size of a floor and the building footprint to develop early (predesign) construction cost estimates. An additional 20–30 percent (or a factor of 1.20–1.30) is generally used to arrive at an estimate for the *floor gross square feet* (FGSF) that accounts for the common areas on the floor. To estimate the total *building gross square feet* (BGSF), an additional 8–12 percent (or a factor of 1.08–1.12) may be required to allow for major mechanical spaces and a central power plant, depending on the scope of the project and existing capacity. Larger factors are required to accommodate unusual design features such as atriums and courtyards. Ultimately, the actual design will determine the final space requirements. However, if the eventual design affords very large net-to-gross space conversion factors and calls for no special architectural features, the overall efficiency of the design should be questioned—for example, look for redundant corridors. Dividing the total BGSF by the actual usable space, or NSF, is often referred to as the *building efficiency ratio* and is expressed as a percentage.

To confuse the matter further, universities often use the term *assignable square feet* to describe all rooms and areas that are available for assignment to an individual program, department, or user. They then use the term *net assignable (or usable) area* to describe the combined total of the NSF and the common or shared areas.

Again, commercial realtors use a slightly different set of terms that need to be understood if a healthcare organization wishes to lease space off campus. The Building Owners and Managers Association International applies the term *usable square feet* to define the footprint of the space that is assigned to the tenant under his direct control and then applies a factor for the tenant's share of the common areas to arrive at the *rentable square feet* on which the tenant will pay rent. In typical multitenant, multistory buildings, the common area factor can range from 14–16 percent. In smaller buildings with fewer amenities and smaller lobbies, the factor ranges from 10–12 percent. The International Facilities Management Association has developed its own definition of rentable square feet that is also used by facility managers to allocate or charge back square footage to specific departments.

Although this discussion of net and gross space may seem tedious, misunderstandings among members of the planning team can be disastrous because the DGSF is typically 20–50 percent higher than the DNSF. For example, confusing department *net* square feet with department *gross* square feet can deem certain facility configuration options feasible when they are not or can result in inaccurate early cost estimates. Physicians and clinical department managers may ask their peers at other institutions for comparative space information and receive the "square feet" with no indication of how it was calculated and may then use this information to demand that their existing space be enlarged. Knowledge of how facility planners calculate space also eliminates surprises when leasing space offsite. NSF and DGSF used for facility planning should also not be confused with other methods of space measurement used by finance departments to account for charge backs to individual departments, cost reimbursement, asset tracking, and so on.

## BED ALLOCATION AND ORGANIZATION

Any facility assessment of an acute care hospital should begin with an inventory and analysis of the inpatient nursing units. Inpatient nursing units are modular in design and vary in the number and type of patient rooms (private, semiprivate), configuration of the patient toilet and bathing facilities, and the total DGSF used to support the specific number of beds. The following data should be collected for each inpatient nursing unit:

- Bed licensure by category of beds, acuity, or service line, according to the specific state regulatory requirements
- Current number of staffed inpatient beds on which the daily or monthly census and occupancy are calculated
- Number of staffed beds in private rooms versus double or semiprivate rooms (or multiple-bed rooms)
- Total number of staffed patient rooms by nursing unit, including private and multiple-bed rooms

In addition, the *design capacity* of each nursing unit should be identified on the basis of physical inspection of the unit, current architectural drawings, or both. The design capacity refers to the total number of beds that could be deployed for inpatient care with minimal renovation, regardless of the number of beds actually staffed at any given time. Additional beds and rooms that may be counted as part of the design capacity may include patient rooms temporarily used as offices or storage rooms (but where the headwalls and utilities are still intact) or smaller, semiprivate rooms used as private rooms during low-census periods. The nursing units should be further aggregated by the type of beds they contain—for example, general medical/surgical, intensive care, maternity, or psychiatric. This breakdown helps the planning team to understand which beds are generally interchangeable in such a way that they can be readily reassigned from one service line to another versus those that are designed as unique units for a specific patient population. Additional information on evaluating inpatient bed capacity is provided in chapter 5 along with an example of an inpatient bed inventory (see exhibit 5.2).

## SPACE LOCATION AND CONFIGURATION

With a thorough understanding of the various types of space in a healthcare facility, one of the key steps in developing a facility planning database is to document the functional layout of your current facilities by identifying where different categories of space are located. Simple floor plans that identify department locations by floor, building, or wing need to be assembled, as shown in exhibit 2.3. Most organizations have as-is architectural drawings in an electronic format, which can be used to delineate existing department boundaries. The newly generated department location or *block* floor plans are typically color coded according to the category of space and are reduced to a manageable size. Building section, or "stacking," diagrams (as shown in exhibit 2.4), are also useful communication tools.

**Exhibit 2.3 Example: Department Location Diagram (Floor Plan)**

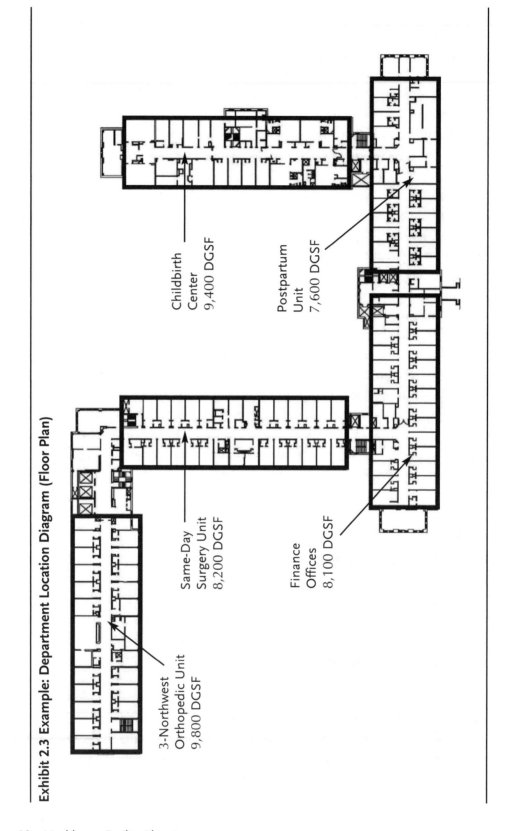

Childbirth Center
9,400 DGSF

Postpartum Unit
7,600 DGSF

Same-Day Surgery Unit
8,200 DGSF

Finance Offices
8,100 DGSF

3-Northwest Orthopedic Unit
9,800 DGSF

**Exhibit 2.3 Example: Department Location Diagram (Floor Plan)**

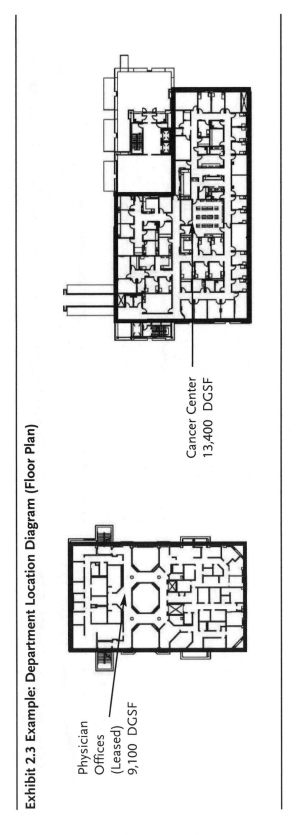

Physician
Offices
(Leased)
9,100 DGSF

Cancer Center
13,400 DGSF

## Exhibit 2.4 Example: Building Section Diagram

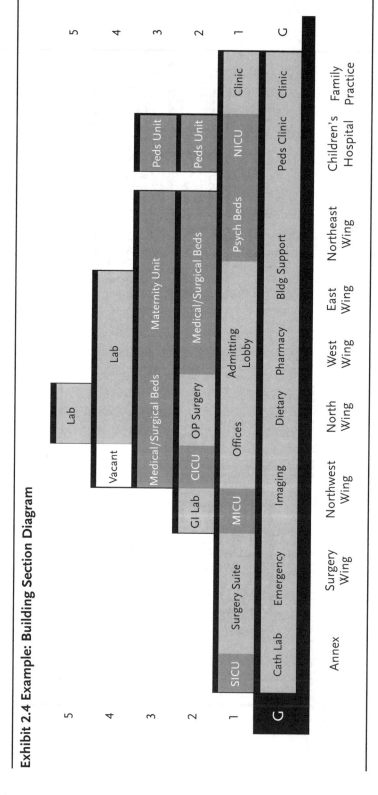

## MAJOR DIAGNOSTIC AND TREATMENT SPACES

In addition to the number of staffed beds, an inventory of major diagnostic and treatment spaces will be key to evaluating your current facility capacity (addressed in chapter 5). The major diagnostic and treatment spaces—rooms, cubicles, or open stretcher bays—that generate revenue and affect the workload and that can be accommodated at your organization include the following:

- ED treatment rooms or bays
- Surgical operating rooms—such as general, open heart, and other specialty rooms—and patient preparation bays and recovery bays
- Labor, delivery, operating, and caesarian section rooms and recovery spaces
- Diagnostic imaging procedure rooms such as X-ray, computed tomography, and magnetic resonance imaging
- Interventional procedure rooms such as cardiac catheterization and angiography
- Other procedure rooms with fixed equipment such as endoscopy and radiation oncology units
- Exam and procedure rooms with mobile equipment such as ultrasound, echocardiography, and electrocardiography machines
- Exam and treatment rooms, typically found in clinics
- Other procedure, treatment, or recovery bays typically used for chemotherapy, medical procedures, and physical therapy

For major imaging and interventional procedure rooms, the current type of equipment and its acquisition date should be identified. As is discussed in chapter 5, the age and sophistication of the equipment may have a significant impact on its capacity to handle a given workload.

## SPACE ALLOCATION

Having two architects or facility managers measure the same building and arrive at the same net and gross square footage numbers is virtually impossible unless they agree on the method of measurement and a clear definition of what is included and excluded, as described previously. Using computer-aided drafting supported by field measurements is far more accurate than trying to scale from old architectural drawings that may not reflect as-is versus as-built conditions. Once the floor plans are in an electronic format, the footprint of each department can be electronically defined and measured. The resulting inventory of current DGSF can then be organized by major functional category of space and the space tabulated by department, floor level, and building as appropriate.

Exhibit 2.5 shows the typical distribution of assignable space (DGSF) in a community hospital (excluding physician practice space) according to my experience in the field. The ranges represent variations in patient accommodations (private vs. semiprivate inpatient room mix); service consolidation versus decentralization; on-site versus off-site service locations; and institutional policies regarding the scope of patient, visitor, and staff amenities.

Why all the emphasis on these functional categories of space? There are two primary reasons. First, organizing space in this manner facilitates cost-effective space reconfiguration, because the space occupied by a department in a functional category can be more readily and cost-effectively redeployed for use by another department in that category. Second, the grouping of departments that have similar facility requirements often exposes new opportunities for the sharing of space between organizational entities.

The DGSF for an inpatient nursing unit should include the eight-foot circulation corridors in the nursing units, though they are used for public egress. However, central elevator lobbies, elevator banks, stairwells, and major mechanical space should be excluded from the DGSF for an inpatient nursing unit.

**Exhibit 2.5 Typical Community Hospital Space Allocation (DGSF)**

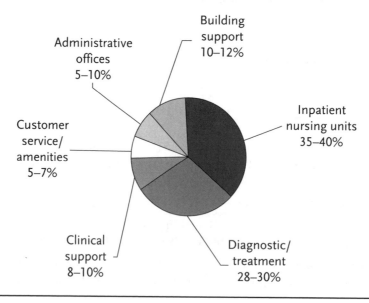

## MAJOR PHYSICAL PLANT AND INFRASTRUCTURE ISSUES

First, let's address how information about the condition of the physical plant and building infrastructure is used during the facility master planning process. The primary reason for a detailed engineering evaluation is to identify code noncompliance and other critical physical plant issues that could affect the viability of the business enterprise. Second, for capital budgeting, infrastructure deficiencies must be identified and costs and a timetable developed for their correction. Every healthcare organization should include the ongoing upgrading of its infrastructure and physical plant as one of its long-range facility investment strategies. Like any other business, healthcare organizations need to continually maintain and update their physical plants and retool their facilities to meet changing demand and integrate new technology. The ongoing cost of infrastructure upgrading must be known while other construction or reconfiguration costs are identified. This planning ensures that adequate dollars are available for both over the multiyear planning period.

Physical plant and infrastructure upgrading issues are more or less critical to the facility master planning effort, depending on the general age and condition of a medical center's facilities. An exhaustive and comprehensive engineering assessment may be undertaken that incorporates a detailed evaluation of all elements of the physical plant, including structural, mechanical, plumbing, electrical, and fire safety systems. However, healthcare organizations should be cautious when embarking on this type of comprehensive and detailed assessment of the physical plant before they undertake a thorough analysis of the current functional layout, wayfinding issues, and future space need. Buildings and wings have a tendency to become functionally obsolete for specific services before they become physically obsolete, and time and money may be saved if a more specific and targeted engineering assessment will suffice.

Hospital boards may face sticker shock when the results of an extensive engineering assessment are presented and the associated costs itemized. Such estimates can be particularly distressing because the benefit of spending millions of dollars on infrastructure upgrading is not generally apparent to patients, physicians, and staff. Some board members may recall that the construction of the original hospital had cost less than the current dollars requested for a new power plant, electrical upgrading, elevator replacement, fire safety improvements, and the like. This memory frequently results in the question of how much replacing the existing hospital with new construction would cost in lieu of spending so much money on upgrading the infrastructure.

# SUMMARY OF BASELINE FACILITY PLANNING DATA

The following list summarizes the baseline facility planning data that are needed:

- Site plan that includes property boundaries, campus circulation routes, parking by type, and key building entrance points
- Department block floor plans
- Summary of inpatient beds and nursing units
- Identification of major diagnostic and treatment spaces as well as the type and age of imaging equipment applicable
- Space inventory in DGSF
- Identification of major infrastructure issues and remediation costs

## REFERENCE

Facilities Guidelines Institute. 2014. *Guidelines for Design and Construction of Hospitals and Outpatient Facilities*. Chicago: American Society for Healthcare Engineering of the American Hospital Association.

Hayward, C. 2015. *SpaceMed Guide: A Space Planning Guide for Healthcare Facilities*, 3rd ed. Ann Arbor, MI: HA Ventures.

# CHAPTER 3

# Defining Strategic Direction and Future Demand

IN THE THIRD edition of *Healthcare Strategic Planning*, author Alan M. Zuckerman (2012) describes a four-stage strategic planning approach for healthcare organizations:

1. *Environmental assessment* involves a review of the organization's mission, philosophy, and culture; an external assessment of the market structure and dynamics; an internal assessment of distinctive characteristics; and an evaluation of competitive position in the market.
2. *Organizational direction* is where mission, vision, alternative futures, and key strategies are formulated.
3. *Strategy formulation* is where goals and objectives for the organization are established, particularly related to critical issues.
4. *Implementation planning* involves identifying the actions needed to implement the plan, such as the schedule, priorities, and resources.

The first stage focuses on the question, where are we now? The second and third stages address the question, where should we be going? The fourth stage responds to the question, how do we get there? Although this overall process is similar to that used to develop a long-range facility master plan (or capital investment strategy), most healthcare organizations use the term *strategic planning* to describe market planning with an increasing emphasis on surviving financially while fulfilling the organization's mission. The strategic (market) planning process logically precedes facility planning, assuming that business strategies must be in place and future demand must be forecasted before resources—such as facilities, equipment, and staff—can be defined. However, there are several benefits to integrating, or at least overlapping, these efforts.

## UNDERSTANDING YOUR MARKET AND PATIENT POPULATION

An important component of strategic planning is an assessment of the organization's market and the socioeconomic characteristics of the service area population. Patients may have different perceptions and expectations depending on their age, gender, ethnicity, average income, education level, occupation, and so on. Although the patient population to be served by a healthcare organization may change over the life of the facility, hospital leaders, facility planners, and architects should have a general understanding of the patient population for which their facilities are planned.

## INTEGRATING FACILITY PLANNING WITH STRATEGIC (MARKET) PLANNING

Integrating the facility assessment with the internal market assessment during the strategic planning process brings a new dimension to this effort. For example, a review of facility strengths and weaknesses, along with potential facility and equipment capacity constraints and surpluses, may reveal unforeseen opportunities for the organization to embark on new strategies with minimal risk. Alternately, the organization may decide early in the process to discard specific strategies that are deemed cost prohibitive.

Specifically, surplus space and equipment, such as a vacant nursing unit or excess surgical capacity, may provide quick and low-risk opportunities to launch a new program or cultivate an existing one with minimal capital investment. On the other hand, if an organization must construct and equip new space, the financial risk and the delayed timing could render a particular strategy less desirable.

If an organization is faced with a deteriorating physical plant that requires millions of dollars of infrastructure upgrading just to stay in business, then its strategic planning efforts may be focused on revenue growth and financial viability.

## BRIDGING THE GAP: UTILIZATION ANALYSES THAT ARE UNIQUE TO FACILITY PLANNING

Strategic plans for healthcare organizations vary in the degree to which specific strategies and actions are translated into quantified demand forecasts and tangible resource requirements such as facilities, equipment, and staff. A gap often exists between the implementation planning stage that concludes the strategic planning process and the input needed to commence the facility planning process. The translation of the organization's strategic planning initiatives and future service volumes into clinical service needs by location and corresponding space requirements is a critical aspect of facility master planning. Whether developed as part of the strategic planning process or as part of the facility planning process, identification of the following, at a minimum, is required:

- New programs and services that will require space or new facilities
- Future bed need by clinical service line, acuity, patient accommodation type, and location, including the development of "high bed" and "low bed" scenarios (if applicable)
- Ambulatory services strategy relative to projected demand, service delivery locations, and physician office needs
- Future ancillary workload projections (by location) for selected diagnostic and treatment services, with inpatient and outpatient breakdown

Strategies related to market penetration, physician recruitment, and customer satisfaction, along with other studies on the current status and future direction of key clinical service lines, should also be incorporated into the facility planning effort. In particular, detailed business plans for new or expanding clinical service lines provide a sound foundation for facility planning.

Even though analyses of current and historical inpatient utilization, bed need, and ancillary workload projections are commonly undertaken as part of the strategic planning process, planning a facility requires a different perspective.

## HIGH BED AND LOW BED SCENARIOS

For facility planning purposes, projecting the need for an absolute number of beds at some future date is not nearly as important as identifying the range of beds required on the basis of the most optimistic and pessimistic views of future market conditions. This type of sensitivity analysis can help an organization understand the impact of forecasting inaccuracies. Such awareness is particularly important because decisions to expand or replace inpatient facilities start a chain reaction of events and involve a significant commitment of dollars, staff time, and operational disruption.

Considering the fluctuation in demand for inpatient beds over the past several decades, as described in chapter 1, hospitals now face a series of confusing choices.

As mentioned in chapter 1, after the advent in the 1980s of Medicare's diagnosis-related group (DRG) payment methodology in the public sector and managed care in the private sector, healthcare strategists and policy experts advised hospitals to reduce their surplus inpatient bed capacity as admissions, use rates, and lengths of stay declined. Hospitals reacted with downsizings, consolidations, and closures, effectively reducing inpatient capacity, though the decline slowed after 2003. Inpatient admissions in the United States rose between 1992 to 2012; however, both the rate of inpatient admissions and the average length of stay have reached the lowest levels on record, creating an overall decline in the demand for inpatient beds (American Hospital Association and Avalere Health 2014). The Affordable Care Act encourages the management of population health across the care continuum in an effort to keep patients healthy—and out of acute care facilities—through preventive and primary care services. Though the needs of aging baby boomers and the newly insured continue to grow, inpatient utilization may continue to decline thanks to sophisticated diagnostics, minimally invasive treatment, and the shift from a hospital-centric to a population-centric model.

High bed and low bed need scenarios can be modeled by varying future planning assumptions relative to use rate, market share, length of stay, and occupancy rate (shown in exhibit 3.1). Any one or all of these variables can be modified to develop a realistic range of future bed need for a specific organization. The goal of this type of analysis is to evaluate the magnitude of renovation or construction necessary given the range of optimistic versus pessimistic scenarios as illustrated in the case study presented in chapter 12.

Historically, 80 percent occupancy was used as a target for acute medical and surgical nursing units. However, organizations with all private patient rooms are reevaluating this target. Given the high cost of construction, as well as planning uncertainties, many financial officers are willing to accept the risk of not accommodating all demand during peak periods in lieu of having vacant patient rooms during average census periods. Statistically, a hospital with all private patient rooms should be able to maintain a higher occupancy rate than one with a large number of semiprivate or multiple-bed rooms. Targeting a higher occupancy level is not practical for an organization with a high percentage of semiprivate patient rooms.

Target occupancy rates for an individual nursing unit or service line are generally a function of the nature of arrivals (random vs. predictable), the inherent risk of not accommodating peak demand (intensive care vs. behavioral health), the size of the service or unit, and seasonal fluctuations in demand. These factors are why intensive care, obstetric, and pediatric units may be planned with much lower target occupancy rates (such as 70 percent) and behavioral health units may be planned with higher rates (such as 95 percent).

**Exhibit 3.1 Comparison of Future Bed Need Scenarios**

| | Current | Future Bed Need Scenarios | | |
|---|---|---|---|---|
| | | Low Bed Need (Declining Market Share) | Medium Bed Need (Current Market Share) | High Bed Need (Increased Market Share) |
| Service-area population | 445,030 | 490,000 | 490,000 | 490,000 |
| Use rate (admissions/1,000) | 113.5 | 113.5 | 113.5 | 113.5 |
| Hospital market share | 27.4% | 26.1% | 27.4% | 30.1% |
| Hospital admissions | 13,840 | 14,516 | 15,239 | 16,740 |
| Hospital length of stay | 5.40 | 4.90 | 5.15 | 5.40 |
| Hospital average daily census | 205 | 195 | 215 | 248 |
| Bed need at: | | | | |
| 90% occupancy | | 217 | 239 | 276 |
| 85% occupancy | | 229 | 253 | 292 |
| 80% occupancy | | 244 | 269 | 310 |
| Current bed capacity | 240 | 240 | 240 | 240 |
| Bed surplus (+) or deficit (−) | | +23 to −4 | −1 to −29 | −36 to −70 |

## EVALUATING BED SCENARIOS WHEN THERE IS A DEFICIT OF PRIVATE PATIENT ROOMS

The trend in planning acute care hospitals is toward providing only private patient rooms and eliminating multiple-bed rooms or wards. If your facility was constructed with only private rooms, then you can skip to the next section. Otherwise, you will be challenged with planning a staged conversion of semiprivate rooms to privates over time. However, such changes may offer you additional flexibility that could offset forecasting inaccuracies. If the low bed scenario plays out, then some of the existing semiprivate rooms could be used as single occupancy. On the other hand, if the high bed scenario comes to fruition, then the organization could deploy some of the rooms as semiprivates during peak census periods.

Hospitals can achieve maximum flexibility by providing private, acuity adaptable patient rooms that can be used to deliver varying levels of care. Single rooms maximize the patient's privacy, minimize costly patient transfers, facilitate the participation of family members in care, and better address special needs such as infection control.

Although higher occupancy levels are achievable in units with only private rooms, the associated construction costs will increase slightly because of increased space requirements and additional patient toilet and bathing facilities. Thus, because of budgetary or existing facility constraints, in some cases planning for a mixture of private and semiprivate patient rooms may be necessary (see exhibit 3.2). Although semiprivate rooms are less costly to construct, they are also less flexible and more beds are needed to accommodate a given average daily census than in an all private room scenario because of the need to separate male and female patients and those with incompatible medical conditions. Some organizations pursue a prudent approach by planning enough total patient "rooms" to accommodate the average daily census in such a way that semiprivate rooms are deployed only during high-census periods—such as when the census is above 85 percent occupancy.

## SAME-DAY-STAY PATIENTS AND OBSERVATION BEDS

The forecasting of beds that are used for observation, with a length of stay generally less than 24 hours, also varies from one organization to the next. Patients requiring observation may be held in the emergency department (ED) or placed on a traditional inpatient nursing unit for a 23-hour stay or, in the case of Medicare patients, for fewer than two midnights of medically necessary

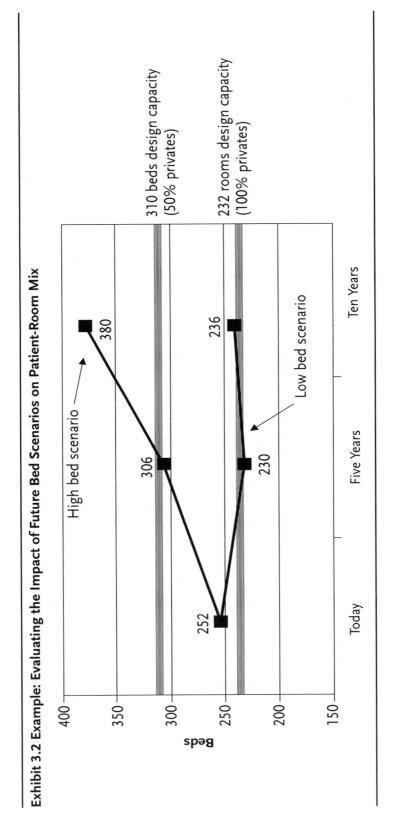

Exhibit 3.2 Example: Evaluating the Impact of Future Bed Scenarios on Patient-Room Mix

hospital care. Observation patients are frequently housed on inpatient nursing units, affecting inpatient bed capacity. Observation status is primarily used for reimbursement purposes; the "outpatient" and his care may vary little from that of a traditional inpatient.

Nursing staff will often take issue with bed forecasts that fail to account for this growing group of patients that typically occupy inpatient beds. Although recording these patients on daily census reports is becoming more common for healthcare organizations, most traditional bed need methodologies are not designed to accommodate this group of patients. At the minimum, the current daily number of observation and same-day patients occupying an inpatient bed should be estimated on the basis of central data sources or by conducting periodic data sampling unit by unit. With these data, the optimal setting for these patients should be identified—for example, inpatient bed, same-day medical procedure unit, observation unit, or the ED—and future assumptions regarding bed need by location (setting) can be confirmed.

## LOCATION, LOCATION, LOCATION

The real estate investment mantra "location, location, location" is critical when assessing and projecting healthcare utilization data for facility planning. Healthcare organizations collect data for many different purposes, most notably for financial accounting of revenue and costs. Data may also be used to evaluate operational efficiency and staff productivity. For facility planning purposes, however, utilization data by location are most critical. Such data are often difficult to ascertain from the forecasts of inpatient and ancillary service demand generated for a strategic plan.

Emergency visits and obstetrics deliveries (births) are often projected during the strategic planning process by applying use rates per 1,000 population and market-share assumptions to forecast future (market-based) demand. However, the rigor of forecasting other ancillary workloads is often insufficient. Forecasts for major services—including surgical cases, endoscopies, imaging procedures, and invasive and noninvasive cardiology—are often developed by department or service line managers (a bottom-up approach). A typical methodology involves simply extending the historical trend forward to the designated future planning horizon. Inpatient and outpatient breakdowns may not even be delineated. The forecasting of less traditional service volumes—such as hospital-based medical procedures, including transfusions, biopsies, and IV therapy—is often even less scientific.

Procedure volumes gathered from central data sources do not typically designate the location that the procedures were performed, although department statistics are generally more detailed. Procedures performed at the point of care with portable equipment are often grouped with department-based inpatient or outpatient procedures. This categorization is a particular problem with routine radiology, fluoroscopy, electrocardiogram, and ultrasound statistics, where procedures performed with portable equipment at the patient's bedside or in an outpatient clinic may represent a sizable proportion of the workload.

In general, ancillary workloads should be broken down into inpatient and outpatient components, and each should be projected separately. The inpatient component can be correlated to inpatient admissions by analyzing the historical ratio per admission and then applying a target ratio to the forecasted admissions. Projection of the outpatient component is far less scientific and should be qualitatively based on market strategy, physician recruitment plans, pending reimbursement changes, and historical trends. Exhibit 3.3 provides an example for forecasting surgery, computed tomography (CT), and magnetic resonance imaging (MRI) workloads.

Overly optimistic growth projections prepared by department or service line managers should be challenged, particularly if they result in a decision to commit capital dollars to additional equipment, procedure rooms, and support space. Also, outpatient volumes that are erratic and show no discernible trend should be monitored. In some cases, current workloads may be artificially low because of problems recruiting qualified staff. Knowledge of individual physicians and their status should also be incorporated into the projection of outpatient volumes. Examples may include

- surgeons who lack commitment to the organization and alternate between hospital-based and outpatient surgery facilities year to year or who are planning to invest in their own freestanding ambulatory surgery center;
- cardiologists who alternate between competing organizations depending on which facility has the latest technology; and
- physicians whose interest in performing specific procedures such as X-ray, endoscopy, and chemotherapy at the hospital-based facility, versus in their own offices, fluctuates depending on reimbursement and regulatory issues.

Highly productive physicians or surgeons who are close to retirement may also have a significant impact on future workload projections. Alternately, physician recruitment plans that could result in substantial workload growth should be factored into workload forecasts. Unfortunately, I have seen many instances in which a physician

**Exhibit 3.3 Example: Projecting Ancillary Workloads**

| Med/Surg/ICU | 2012 | 2013 | 2014 | 2015 | | 2020 | Comments |
|---|---|---|---|---|---|---|---|
| Admissions | 26,578 | 27,165 | 28,423 | 29,375 | ↑ | 41,000 | Projected medical/surgical/ICU admissions |

| Surgery | 2012 | 2013 | 2014 | 2015 | | 2020 | |
|---|---|---|---|---|---|---|---|
| Open-heart cases | 1,288 | 1,303 | 1,334 | 1,296 | ↑ | 1,296 | Status quo assumed |
| Other IP cases | 10,465 | 10,974 | 11,657 | 12,349 | | 17,220 | Calculated |
| IP cases/admissions | 0.39 | 0.40 | 0.41 | 0.42 | | 0.42 | Assumes current ratio will be maintained |
| OP cases | 13,984 | 15,893 | 16,716 | 16,901 | | 17,000 | Will level off with off-site competition |
| % OP cases | 54% | 56% | 56% | 55% | | 48% | Calculated |
| **Total cases** | 25,737 | 28,170 | 29,707 | 30,546 | | 35,516 | |

| CT | 2012 | 2013 | 2014 | 2015 | | 2020 | |
|---|---|---|---|---|---|---|---|
| IP tests | 9,350 | 10,220 | 11,519 | 12,169 | ↑ | 16,810 | Calculated |
| IP tests/admissions | 0.35 | 0.38 | 0.41 | 0.41 | | 0.41 | Assumes current ratio will be maintained |
| OP tests | 17,410 | 21,187 | 22,788 | 23,980 | | 27,800 | Assumes growth of 3 percent per year |
| % OP tests | 65% | 67% | 66% | 66% | | 62% | Calculated |
| **Total tests** | 26,760 | 31,407 | 34,307 | 36,149 | | 44,610 | |

| MRI | 2012 | 2013 | 2014 | 2015 | | 2020 | |
|---|---|---|---|---|---|---|---|
| IP tests | 2,107 | 2,256 | 2,294 | 2,456 | ↑ | 3,280 | Calculated |
| IP tests/admissions | 0.08 | 0.08 | 0.08 | 0.08 | | 0.08 | Assumes current ratio will be maintained |
| OP tests | 5,910 | 5,822 | 6,005 | 6,320 | | 8,060 | Assumes growth of 5 percent per year |
| % OP tests | 74% | 72% | 72% | 72% | | 71% | Calculated |
| **Total tests** | 8,017 | 8,078 | 8,299 | 8,776 | | 11,340 | |

specialist demanded new equipment and space from a trusting hospital administrator and then skipped across town to the competing hospital once the first hospital's new facilities opened.

## PLANNING CENTERS OF EXCELLENCE

For a special situation in which an organization is planning to realign and colocate specific treatments and procedures by service line, it may be challenged when identifying and quantifying the specific workloads that will occur in the new center of excellence. Exercise caution so that projected workloads are not counted twice, resulting in the planning of capacity at both a new specialty center and an existing hospital-based department or freestanding diagnostic facility.

## LINKING THE CAPACITY ASSESSMENT TO FORECASTS OF FUTURE DEMAND

Incorporating the capacity assessment described in chapter 5 into the workload forecasting effort is important. In the capacity assessment, the current capacity of each major clinical service is identified on the basis of the existing number of procedure rooms, the equipment and technology, and the specific operational characteristics; then the optimal capacity that could be achieved through operational changes, such as extended hours of operation, new equipment, and procedural changes, is defined. With this knowledge in hand, the workload forecasting activity can be focused on those services that are presently at capacity or near capacity relative to projected future workload volumes.

For example, the planner may determine that an existing surgery suite where 70 percent of the cases are ambulatory, is averaging 750 annual cases per operating room (three cases per day, 250 days per year), which is very low utilization. If weekday hours were extended in such a way that one more case were added each day, the existing number of operating rooms could accommodate a 33 percent increase in workload. In this case, future workload forecasts would not need to be scrutinized unless explosive growth (beyond 33 percent) is anticipated. As another example, if an older CT unit, which accommodates 12–16 patients in an eight-hour shift, is replaced with a high-speed model that can accommodate 16–22 patients per shift, the unit could achieve a 35 percent increase in workload without facility expansion. If the same imaging suite were also able to staff and schedule patients for six hours on Saturdays, the hospital could accommodate future growth of more than

50 percent. With this kind of operational flexibility, facility planners need spend little time debating the accuracy of forecasts.

## THE APPROPRIATE PLANNING HORIZON FOR FACILITY PLANNING

Much debate often takes place regarding appropriate planning horizons. Population-based forecasts of inpatient admissions, births, or ED visits must correspond with the planning horizons of the available population projections and will only be as accurate as the population forecasts on which they are based. At the same time, new healthcare facilities built today must meet the needs of patients for many decades beyond the standard five- to ten-year strategic planning horizon. A prudent approach is first to understand the current and optimal capacity of existing equipment, procedure rooms, and support space and then to focus on those services for which capacity is an issue. Finally, as discussed in chapter 15, the planning of flexible, multiuse, or adaptable facilities can cost-effectively offset inaccuracies in workload forecasting. Unless a new or replacement healthcare facility is being planned, most healthcare organizations will translate their facility development strategies into immediate (within two years), short-term (within two to five years), and long-range (beyond five years) projects, as described in chapter 7. This approach is necessary because of the length of the planning, design, and construction cycle and the capital funding and staff energy required to execute the facility master plan.

## REFERENCES

American Hospital Association and Avalere Health. 2014. *TrendWatch Chartbook 2014: Trends Affecting Hospitals and Health Systems*. Accessed January 13, 2016. www.aha.org/research/reports/tw/chartbook/2014/14chartbook.pdf.

Zuckerman, A. M. 2012. *Healthcare Strategic Planning*, 3rd ed. Chicago: Health Administration Press.

# CHAPTER 4

# Coordinating Operations Improvement Initiatives and Planned Technology Investments with Facility Planning

To OPTIMIZE YOUR capital investments, facility planning should be integrated with institution-wide and service line–specific operations improvement initiatives and also coordinated with planned information technology (IT) investments. This integrated approach provides an opportunity for facility reconfiguration or expansion to potentially improve operational efficiency, enhance customer service, and provide future operational flexibility. Coordinating an organization's IT strategic planning efforts with long-range facility planning may offer new opportunities to unbundle current space and may improve the accuracy of the capital budgeting process. For example, assumptions regarding future capital outlays for computer hardware should be coordinated with long-range strategies regarding the functional use and future status of specific buildings or facility components, such as a change in functional use or demolition.

## INSTITUTION-WIDE OPERATIONS IMPROVEMENT INITIATIVES

The objective of most of the operations reengineering efforts in which I have been involved since the mid-1990s was to reduce the number of hospital departments and increase the span of control—for example, increasing the number of subordinates per manager or supervisor. Many departments were operating more or less autonomously, focused on their own bottom lines. From my experience, consolidation of traditional hospital departments through operations reengineering has done the following:

- Improved the continuity and quality of care with a more integrated provider team
- Enhanced productivity through the cross-training of staff

- Improved customer service and facilitated wayfinding with one-stop shopping
- Generally provided more efficient use of staff, equipment, and space

The ongoing movement toward patient-centered care responds to the need to redesign the patient care delivery system in such a way that the hospital resources and personnel are organized around the patient rather than specialized departments. The trend toward decentralization of many modalities to the point of care—for example, laboratory testing, imaging, and admitting—further challenges rigid departmental boundaries, organizational structures, and job descriptions.

What does this shift have to do with the facility planning process? In the traditional facility planning approach, the facility planner or programmer solicits input from individual department managers and their staff, which often results in the replication of existing, inefficient organizational structures and operational systems at a time when hospitals can seize the tremendous opportunity to use facility reconfiguration as the impetus to effect operational change. Department leadership may be unaware of best practices occurring elsewhere, or it may be reluctant to challenge the status quo. Multidisciplinary task forces, focused on specific patient processes, may help department managers to think outside of the box. However, strong administrative leadership and participation is needed if organization structures are to be altered or if job descriptions are to be revised. Some organizations may not have the resources (or the energy) to embark on significant operations restructuring during predesign planning. Regardless, planning and designing selected staff workstations and procedure rooms contiguous with each other, in such a way that staff from different departments work side by side, may eventually facilitate more formal operations reorganization and cross-training of staff.

## COMMON INSTITUTION-WIDE SYSTEMS AND RELATED TECHNOLOGY

An understanding of common institution-wide operational systems, processes, and related technology in current use is critical to a successful facility planning effort. Specifically, facility planners need to identify current operational problems, priorities, and operations improvement opportunities related to the following:

- Customer expectations
- Departments exhibiting operational problems, particularly relating to multiple-site or divided operations

- ◆ Effectiveness of common institution-wide systems and related technology that affect resource use, such as staffing, equipment, and space:
  - – Wayfinding and orientation, outpatient registration, scheduling, and test-result reporting to referring physicians
  - – Inpatient admitting, discharge, billing, and collections
  - – Health information management (health records)
  - – Patient transportation
- ◆ Materials and supply chain management
- ◆ Departments perceived as having major facility deficiencies with regard to inappropriate space allocation and functional relationships, which affect operational efficiency
- ◆ Equipment or technology constraints and anticipated improvements
- ◆ Recent developments, trends, and operations improvement initiatives that will significantly affect facility needs

Once documented, assumptions regarding future changes can then be incorporated into the facility planning process.

## CLINICAL SERVICE LINE OPERATIONS IMPROVEMENT INITIATIVES

Facility planners should review operations improvement initiatives for specific clinical service lines such as emergency, surgery, and imaging and incorporate appropriate operational assumptions into assessments of capacity and workload throughput as part of the facility planning process. If successfully implemented, such operational improvements may have a dramatic effect on the need for exam and treatment spaces, overall space, and ultimately construction costs. Exhibit 4.1 illustrates the relationship between emergency department (ED) performance, as measured by treatment space turnaround time, and the number of annual visits that can be accommodated in each treatment space.

## ADVANCES IN INFORMATION AND COMMUNICATIONS TECHNOLOGY

As noted in chapter 1, the healthcare industry will increasingly rely on data, including electronic health records, financial and management information, imaging

**Exhibit 4.1 Relationship Between ED Performance and Capacity**

| Emergency Department Performance | Average Treatment Space Turnaround Time (Minutes) | Average Annual Visits per Treatment Space |
|---|---|---|
| Poor | 210 | 1,100–1,200 |
| Average | 150 | 1,200–1,600 |
| Best | 120 | 1,600–1,900 |

*Source:* Reprinted from Hayward (2015).

studies, sensor and device readings, voice communications, and telemedicine information. Ongoing advances in information technology, along with new staff positions and job descriptions, are changing historical perceptions regarding necessary functional relationships. Many traditional health and financial data management functions are being consolidated—including medical records maintenance, quality assurance, risk management, infection control, finance, data processing, and telecommunications—as data become increasingly computerized and common databases generate data more quickly and effectively.

Although the healthcare sector has historically lagged behind other industries in the use of information and telecommunications technology, advances in networking and mobile computing are beginning to affect operational efficiency and quality of care. Information systems networks facilitate the delivery, management, and administration of patient care from any setting and allow the sharing of information between and across systems. A network with Internet and intranet functions provides access to medical information from all care settings and requires that disparate, nonintegrated, stand-alone systems—such as radiology departments, pharmacies, laboratories, finance departments, and materials management—be replaced or integrated. Eventually, these networks will also connect to the patient's home. Virtual workplaces and care settings, supported by networks, will result in greater mobility in the workforce and affect the amount, type, and location of space.

## CONSIDERING NEW OPERATIONAL AND FACILITY CONFIGURATION MODELS

By implementing a continuous improvement process, many healthcare organizations challenge traditional, inefficient organizational structures and operational systems on an ongoing basis. However, some of the benefits of reengineering can only be achieved through physical facility reconfiguration. For example, the physical reorganization and consolidation of similar functions enhance operational efficiency, create opportunities for cross-training of staff, and reduce the number of managers and supervisors. These changes may result in a reduction in space need, because a smaller staff requires fewer offices and workstations and quicker throughput lessens the need for expensive procedure rooms and large patient and visitor waiting areas.

New operational models are emerging that not only enhance operational efficiency and optimize the use of scarce resources, such as staff, equipment, and space, but also improve customer service and promote future flexibility. All of these require some degree of facility reconfiguration and should be considered when healthcare leaders explore major facility expansion or replacement.

I have been involved in some of the following new operational models:

- Developing a customer service center
- Consolidating express testing services
- Reconfiguring hospital diagnostic services
- Integrating surgical and imaging procedure space
- Rethinking interventional services
- Developing a medical procedure unit
- Developing an observation unit
- Rethinking the traditional intensive care unit (ICU)
- Planning the laboratory of the future
- Planning the pharmacy of the future
- Creating a generic administrative office suite
- Unbundling building support services
- Rethinking traditional parking lots and structures

These new concepts seldom emerge when a traditional facility planning process is deployed—for example, if the process is led by a designer or architect with input from department silos. Implementation of these concepts requires an enlightened leadership team that is willing to challenge the status quo.

## Developing a Customer Service Center

In the traditional healthcare facility, multiple departments and staff are commonly involved in customer intake, access, and processing activities:

- ◆ Volunteers often provide reception, information dissemination, and wayfinding.
- ◆ Inpatient admitting, outpatient registration, coordination of multiple appointments, and scheduling of follow-up appointments are often performed by one or more departments (such as the admitting department or central outpatient registration) or by separate scheduling systems within individual diagnostic and treatment departments.
- ◆ The finance department often performs cashiering, insurance verification, billing, and financial counseling.
- ◆ Patient amenities may be dispersed with insufficient volume at any given location to warrant fixed staffing or facility upgrading.

This scattered structure typically results in fragmented customer service and complicates wayfinding. Although many of these departments are located on the first floor of the facility, only a few staff members in each department actually have face-to-face interaction with visitors, patients, and their families. The question is, how can an organization better use its staff and its space to enhance operational efficiency and improve customer service?

With the continuing focus on patient-centered care and the emergence of multihospital systems, IT, and reengineering techniques, the trend is to consolidate customer intake, processing, and support services into a single operational unit. Such units are often referred to as a *customer service center*, a *patient service center*, *access services*, or a similar designation. I prefer the term *customer* because it can refer to visitors, family members, employers, payers, physicians, staff, and vendors in addition to the patient.

The customer service center is the primary patient and visitor intake, processing, and communication area for a healthcare facility or campus and also includes centralized patient and visitor amenities as illustrated in exhibit 4.2. The customer service center should be located directly inside the primary entrance to the healthcare complex to serve as the initial access point for visitors and most scheduled patients. This area can also function as a "home base" for family members and visitors who are spending increased time at the facility as more treatments and procedures are performed on a same-day basis. Functional components of the customer service center typically include the following:

- *Central reception, intake, and communication area*, including the entrance vestibule, initial reception and communication station for dissemination of information and orientation, family and visitor lounge, discharge lounge, public toilets, phones, automated teller machine (ATM), Internet kiosk, and other amenities for patients and visitors
- *Patient processing and access services*, including admitting, registration, insurance verification, scheduling, cashiering, billing, financial counseling, discharge planning, physician referral, patient and guest relations, and security
- *Other optional services*, such as a patient resource center, an outpatient or retail pharmacy, coffee shop, gift shop, spiritual or pastoral care, and support space for volunteers

Patients and visitors are spending longer periods at acute care hospitals as more procedures shift from an inpatient stay to a same-day stay with a multiple-hour recovery period. Healthcare organizations recognize the need to provide appropriate amenities for family members and visitors, such as a comfortable family and visitor lounge. Some organizations provide free health screenings, use wall space for ongoing art exhibits, provide entertainment, and offer refreshments using food carts in or near the lounge. With many hospitals experiencing severe bed shortages, discharge lounges are becoming increasingly popular as a way to free inpatient rooms for the next patient while the discharged patient waits for transportation to her home. Other patient- and visitor-support services and amenities may include a gift shop, a coffee shop, an outpatient or retail pharmacy, a chapel or meditation room, public toilet facilities, and an ATM. Durable medical equipment—for example, crutches, canes, and orthotic devices—may be dispensed as part of an outpatient pharmacy. Creating a welcoming and healing environment with enhanced amenities should be considered a necessary part of an organization's marketing strategy.

The healthcare sector is beginning to look to the hospitality sector for solutions to ongoing customer service problems that result from archaic organizational structures and inadequate information systems. For example, when a customer visits a hotel, he is greeted by a central reception desk and a comfortable lobby immediately on entry. At this central reception desk, the customer can receive, or be connected with, any needed services; register, pay bills, get information and directions; make a special request regarding housekeeping services; arrange transportation; or schedule a massage. Yet the healthcare industry requires that its customers visit multiple locations and interact with multiple staff members and fragmented systems, assuming that the customers can first determine the

**Exhibit 4.2 Example: Customer Service Center Concept**

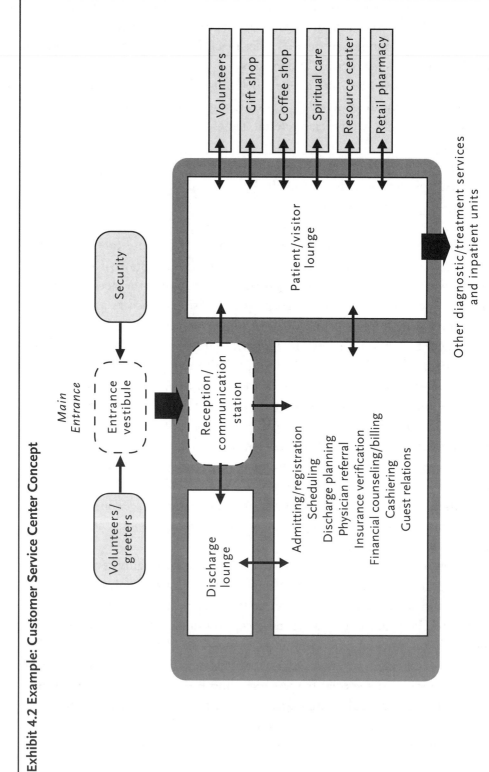

*Source:* Reprinted from Hayward (2015).

appropriate access point for their needed service. The customer service center attempts to replicate the main reception desk typically found in an upscale hotel by using the same hub-and-spoke concept.

## Consolidating Express Testing Services

Healthcare organizations are also consolidating high-volume, quick-turnaround diagnostic services into an express testing center that may be colocated with the customer service center to provide one-stop shopping. These services may include routine blood and urine collection, an electrocardiogram, a chest X-ray, a simple bone X-ray, and preadmission or presurgery consultation. For many acute care hospitals, a significant portion of their outpatient activity involves these routine services, yet patients are often expected to travel to multiple department locations throughout the hospital complex.

As with the customer service center model, the staff work together as a team to provide quality care in an expedient manner. The staff are often cross-trained and report organizationally to a single supervisor rather than to multiple department managers. Patient satisfaction generally improves as healthcare centers simplify wayfinding, expedite patient throughput, decrease waiting times, and improve continuity of care, thus reducing operational costs. Less space is needed on the first floor (prime real estate), and staff not directly involved in face-to-face customer contact are relocated.

Some organizations may choose to locate an *express testing center* adjacent to the lobby of a major medical office building or ambulatory care center to enhance convenience for patients who are simultaneously visiting a physician or to provide more convenient parking and access. However, the key to successful implementation of this concept is to have sufficient use (high volumes) so as not to duplicate resources unnecessarily.

## Reconfiguring Hospital Diagnostic Services

Planning space for diagnostic services, and assessing the need for equipment, can be complicated from many perspectives. Some equipment is becoming miniaturized, portable (even handheld), and more affordable so that it can be easily used at the patient's bedside, in the physician's office, or even in the patient's home. Other equipment has become increasingly specialized, continuing to require a large footprint, unique facility design features, and a big investment. Imaging services no longer reside within the boundaries of the radiology department but instead are provided in many locations throughout the healthcare enterprise—often replacing other testing modalities that once occupied stand-alone departments. The challenge is not only to determine what equipment to purchase but also where to locate it.

Hospitals were traditionally designed with a large central radiology department to provide services to inpatients as well as outpatients. As new diagnostic modalities were developed, each was typically designed with its own "storefront" and dedicated space, resulting in significant space allocated to diagnostic services. During the late 1980s and 1990s, many healthcare organizations developed separate outpatient diagnostic centers, often located in an off-site medical office building. At the same time, the use of large, central diagnostic departments in hospitals by inpatients declined as lengths of stay decreased and more patients were tested prior to admission. The miniaturization and increased mobility of equipment also allowed more testing to be conducted at the point of care. As a result, many hospitals were left with significant surplus capacity—particularly for imaging services.

Today, radiography, fluoroscopy, computed tomography (CT) scan, magnetic resonance imaging (MRI), and ultrasound are routinely provided in an outpatient setting, and mammography is performed almost exclusively outside the hospital. However, the acute care hospital continues to be the nexus for new resource-intensive hybrid imaging technologies and interventional procedures that require a significant investment of dollars and a substantial market share to justify the investment. Some less resource-intensive diagnostics also continue to thrive in the hospital setting because of legislation that limits physician self-referrals, staff shortages, and reimbursement for outpatient services, which deters physicians from competing for outpatient business. To improve responsiveness, some services may be decentralized to the point of care—such as the ED, outpatient clinics, or patient care units—either through the use of portable equipment or the creation of a satellite facility. Radiography, CT, and even MRI are commonly provided in large EDs.

As a result, hospital diagnostic services are being reorganized and reconfigured with flexible space to support today's integrated service models with shared staff, equipment, and space. In small hospitals, designers are creating a single diagnostic center comprising reception, waiting, and preprocedure preparation and postprocedure recovery areas shared by multiple departments. In large medical centers, planners may create separate centers for diagnostic imaging and interventional imaging while other diagnostic services may be located in a shared suite or dedicated space or decentralized.

## Integrating Surgical and Imaging Procedure Space

While surgery is becoming less invasive, medical imaging is becoming more interventional and thus no longer limited to diagnostic procedures. Real-time imaging—using a mobile ultrasound or endoscopy unit or a C-arm—has been a standard part of the operating room for many years. However, the *hybrid operating room*—a revolutionary alternative to the conventional operating room—presents a unique planning challenge. Although the definition can vary, the hybrid operating room has permanently installed equipment such as intraoperative computed tomography (iCT), intraoperative magnetic resonance imaging (iMRI), and fixed C-arms—typically used in conjunction with cardiovascular, thoracic, neurosurgery, spinal, and orthopedic procedures—to enable diagnostic imaging before, during, and after a surgical procedure. This allows the surgeon to assess the effectiveness of the surgery and perform further resections or additional interventions—in a single encounter. Many equipment vendors now offer highly specialized, proprietary imaging systems that are permanently integrated with the operating room.

## Rethinking Interventional Services

Healthcare organizations are also increasingly planning a single interventional suite, often contiguous with the surgery suite, that can be shared by interventional radiologists, cardiologists, and endovascular surgeons in lieu of planning separate catheterization laboratories and angiography rooms in the radiology department. This model provides increased future flexibility as clinical programs and medical staff change over time, which may result in a reduction in the number of total procedure rooms that need to be upgraded or constructed. It also minimizes the amount of space needed for patient reception and intake, family waiting, and patient preparation and recovery. The greatest challenge to this model involves turf issues between interventional radiologists, cardiologists, and endovascular surgeons and the promotion of cardiology and vascular centers of excellence.

## Developing a Medical Procedure Unit

Historically, same-day medical procedures have been scattered throughout the hospital or ambulatory care facility, with redundant patient reception, waiting, preparation, recovery, instrument processing, and treatment spaces. Often, locations were selected to optimize historical reimbursement mechanisms. Some healthcare organizations are consolidating various same-day medical procedures in an area that functions as the equivalent of the same-day surgery center. The destination is often referred to as a *medical procedure unit*. Medical procedures may include endoscopies, bronchoscopies, and similar procedures as well as intravenous (IV) therapy, blood transfusions, infusions, paracentesis and thoracentesis, liver biopsies, and the preparation and recovery of patients undergoing various imaging procedures. This concept, as with others discussed in this chapter, requires new job descriptions and flexible space. The space generally includes a patient reception and family waiting area, several procedure spaces (enclosed rooms and open or partially enclosed treatment bays), patient preparation and recovery cubicles, and related support space. Optimal flexibility can be achieved by colocating the medical procedure unit's recovery bays with one or more ED treatment "pods" in such a way that a block or module of treatment and recovery bays can be cross-used to meet peaks and valleys of demand. The colocation of the medical procedure unit treatment and recovery bays with the same-day surgery recovery area can achieve the same flexibility.

## Developing an Observation Unit

An observation unit is used for the extended observation of short-stay patients to avoid their admission as inpatients. Observation status was formerly for patients whose stay was expected to be fewer than 24 hours. However, Medicare patients can now be held for observation for fewer than two midnights of medically necessary hospital care. Observation patients are frequently housed in inpatient nursing units, which can affect inpatient bed capacity.

Hospitals have begun aggregating these patients in a dedicated observation unit in response to crowded and landlocked emergency departments (EDs) and concerns that care can be expedited when patients are not placed in an inpatient nursing unit and thus are out of sight and out of mind. Although observation units require incremental staff, they do not require the resources of a private patient room with an exterior window and an en suite toilet and bathing room. This less demanding set of requirements allows more flexible facility options for accommodating this new and growing group of patients.

Medicare patients are increasingly designated observation patients, and their numbers rose 88 percent over six years, to 1.8 million in 2012 (Medicare Payment Advisory Commission 2015). At the same time, Medicare hospital admissions stayed about the same. An inpatient admission is now considered appropriate if caretakers expect the patient to need two or more midnights of medically necessary hospital care. If not, the patient's care is considered an outpatient service. Because observation is categorized as outpatient care, these patients may also incur copayments for doctors' fees and hospital services and pay higher charges for routine drugs. Observation patients currently cannot receive Medicare coverage for follow-up care in a skilled nursing facility, which requires that they first spend at least three consecutive days (or through three midnights) as an admitted patient. Thus, observation patients often remain in the ED (impeding efficient throughput) or are placed on an inpatient nursing unit. This trend has fueled interest in developing dedicated observation units that do not need to be built to the same standards as inpatient beds.

## Rethinking the Traditional ICU

ICUs are often undermanaged and fraught with hazards, which can result in less-than-desirable outcomes. They are chronically understaffed and chaotic, with a high turnover rate among staff, who frequently burn out from the pressure. In crisis situations, staff often act on instinct with little systematic training to help them respond as a team and with insufficient technology for them to communicate effectively with each other. Moreover, an ICU is a traumatic environment for a patient's family members, who have traditionally been barred from the unit for all but a couple of hours per day and been given minimal information about their loved one's prognosis. Healthcare organizations are redesigning ICUs to better monitor and care for patients, hiring specialists known as intensivists, improving nurse-staffing ratios, and locating pharmacists in the unit. They also involve families directly, opening the once tightly closed units to visitors for as long as 24 hours per day and providing special messaging services with updates for family members. Some patients also designate a family member as their patient advocate to help monitor the quality of their care and to speak up if anything is overlooked.

Remote patient management of critically ill patients is being successfully implemented in a number of US hospitals in response to shortages in nurses and intensivists and pressures to improve the quality of care. A remote or virtual ICU monitoring center—also referred to as an *eICU*—can monitor multiple ICUs at once from a remote location with real time "telepresence," including the review of clinical documentation and medical images, monitoring of vital signs, and use of digital stethoscopes and high-quality video cameras. Use of a remote patient management system allows scarce nursing and physician-intensivist staff members to be more effectively leveraged around the clock and can provide quicker identification of problems, more rapid intervention, improved outcomes, and lower operational costs. This system also allows rural hospitals improved access to intensive care resources.

## Planning the Laboratory of the Future

Laboratory testing has grown from a manual, hands-on process providing a simple test menu—with staff organized by testing methodology or discipline in multiple small rooms—to an automated, multidisciplinary, high-volume, instrument-centric clinical enterprise. A visit to a hospital laboratory today reveals an array of instruments, often operating with little human intervention. The concurrent proliferation of point-of-care testing, providing immediate results, adds another dimension of complexity to laboratory services planning.

The practice of laboratory medicine will continue to experience revolutionary change as a result of new technology and automation, with instrumentation changing as often as every two months, evolving medical practices, consolidation, an increasing number of waived tests, a focus on safety, and the continual need for flexibility. These factors have already had a significant impact on hospital-based laboratories and will continue to affect their operations over the next decade.

## Planning the Pharmacy of the Future

A high-volume pharmacy today looks more like a sophisticated manufacturing plant than a clinical department. Just about any pharmacy task once performed at a hands-on workstation has been automated. Some large hospitals have automated the entire process, from electronic physician orders to individual patient cassettes ready for cart loading and delivery to the patient care unit. Using bar-code technology, sophisticated software, and automated storage and dispensing systems, robotic arms pick, package, and dispense individual doses of pills; compound sterile preparations; and fill IV syringes and bags. An automated inventory management system keeps track of all the products, and automated pharmacy warehouses provide refrigerated and nonrefrigerated storage and retrieval of medications and supplies. In addition to filling medication orders, autonomous mobile robots are being used to make secure deliveries throughout the hospital. Although automation in the pharmacy requires a significant capital investment, it reduces labor costs, lowers the risk of dispensing errors, optimizes inventory control, and provides better security, among other benefits.

## Creating a Generic Administrative Office Suite

The traditional healthcare facility has many departments involved in the administration and management of the organization in accordance with policies established by the governing board. Most of these central administrative services use generic office space with a mix of private offices, open or partially enclosed cubicles, and open workstations to accommodate different hierarchies of staff as dictated by the organizational structure and peak-shift staffing. Patient traffic to these areas is rare.

With the traditional organization of healthcare institutions into multiple, numerous departments, each with dedicated space and narrowly defined job descriptions, efficient space use was difficult to achieve. Many of these departments were forced to resize their staff in response to cost-containment pressures and changing skill requirements, and vacant offices and workstations were scattered throughout the organization. At times, growing departments would need to compress multiple people into a single office, while shrinking departments had surplus space. Many departments also had dedicated conference rooms, which, though infrequently used, were not available for use by other hospital services.

The trend toward the planning of generic administrative office suites, with a central reception and waiting area and groups of conference rooms, provides the most efficient space use and ensures that space is equitably allocated and distributed among the departments and services that need it at any given time. The intent is to assign offices and workstations according to immediate need, allowing for the flexibility to reassign space on a periodic basis as demand changes. This adaptability prevents staff members from becoming territorial about their space. With more sophisticated information systems, space can still be charged to department or cost-center budgets on the basis of use and conference rooms or classrooms scheduled centrally according to demand.

## Unbundling Building Support Services

Also referred to as *hotel services,* building support services include materials management, central sterile processing, dietary services, and environmental and building maintenance services. Just as the clinical areas of the healthcare organization are undergoing operational reengineering to become more patient centered, building support services are changing to make services available on demand to meet patient needs. New operational concepts ensure the availability of supplies and equipment as needed, the delivery of dietary trays at the proper temperature when the patient is ready, and the completion of housekeeping and building maintenance services at the patient's convenience. Although a kitchen is one of the most expensive areas to build and equip in a medical center, most other building services require less expensive, industrial-type space. In most organizations, these functions can share a common administrative area and staff support facilities.

Because of the high cost of space that is built to acute care hospital standards, building support services are being reconfigured to use less (particularly less expensive) space. Just-in-time delivery and stockless materials management models place the burden of storage on the vendor, and the decentralization of other services to the point of care also reduces the amount of space needed in a large central department. Many of these services could appropriately be located adjacent to, or separate from, the acute care facility in a less expensive building (or service center) connected by a tunnel or an enclosed walkway. Multihospital healthcare systems are finding it less costly to support multiple hospital sites from a centralized service center that is remote from one or more hospital sites.

Unfortunately, many existing hospitals were originally designed to support a much larger number of inpatient beds than are currently staffed. With the shift to outpatient and same-day services that require less intensive building support services, many older facilities have a much larger chassis than currently needed. The typical older hospital was designed with building support services located in the basement or on a subgrade level. Many healthcare facilities today are plagued by a rabbit's warren of underground spaces that have received little upgrading or renovation since the original facility was built. Hospital leaders planning new healthcare facilities today should consider locating building support services in a separate, less costly, adjacent (or attached) building that does not have to be built to the more stringent inpatient building codes.

## Rethinking Traditional Parking Lots and Structures

When it comes to parking, hospitals seem to never have enough. Innovations in design and technology, along with careful planning, can mitigate shortages and improve customer convenience. Because easy and convenient access is a prime indicator of hospital customer satisfaction, more US hospitals are rethinking the expansive asphalt parking lot and dreary concrete parking structure. Hospitals today are constructing customer-friendly parking lots and structures that provide easy access, enhanced wayfinding, and optimal security, along with other amenities. Hospitals with dense, urban campuses have been providing valet parking and shuttle services for several decades to facilitate customer access and address security issues. However, healthcare organizations are rethinking how they provide customer access, convenience, and amenities in their parking lots and structures. New amenities and initiatives include

- parking stalls for carpool vans and recreation vehicles and charging stations for electric cars,
- pay-on-foot systems with card readers,

- real-time automated displays that graphically show parking availability by floor and stall,
- pedestrian walkways and bridges connecting to key elevator banks and stairs,
- better lighting and signage (particularly in response to the aging of the population),
- painting unfinished concrete white, and
- providing visual cues to facilitate wayfinding.

Wayfinding is being improved with new features to help patients and visitors remember where they have parked. These features may include specific themes for each floor level, with pictographs or accent colors. Kiosks may also be located at vertical circulation points where the customer can print out a map indicating the location of her parking space to aid in finding her car.

Aesthetics are also becoming more important, with architects and developers specifying facade enhancements to better blend the parking structure with other hospital buildings or with the natural environment in which it is placed (Hayward 2012). For an additional reference, see Hayward (2015).

## REFERENCES

Hayward, C. 2015. *SpaceMed Guide: A Space Planning Guide for Healthcare Facilities*, 3rd ed. Ann Arbor, MI: HA Ventures.

———. 2012. "Rethinking Traditional Parking Lots and Structures." *SpaceMed Newsletter.* Published Winter. www.spacemed.com/newsletter/news51.html.

Medicare Payment Advisory Commission. 2015. *Report to the Congress: Medicare Payment Policy.* Published March 13. www.medpac.gov/documents/reports /mar2015_entirereport_revised.pdf.

# CHAPTER 5

# Identifying Facility Needs
# and Establishing Priorities

WITH AN UNDERSTANDING of your current situation, future market strategy and projected demand, and potential operations improvement opportunities and technology investments, current and future facility needs can be identified and priorities established. The first step is to determine your space needs by location on a department (or service line) basis so that you know the magnitude of current and future space shortages. Other facility deficiencies can then be identified, summarized, and prioritized. Key questions include the following:

◆ How well do we orient our customers as they arrive on the campus and circulate through our facilities?
◆ What is the workload capacity of our current facilities?
◆ Do we have enough space to support our current and projected number of licensed and staffed beds, procedure rooms, equipment, staff, and other required functions?
◆ Is our space organized and configured appropriately?

## UNDERSTANDING THE SPACE PLANNING PROCESS

Space planning typically requires varying levels of detail at different points in the facility planning process. During the facility master planning stage, a broad-brush approach is used to assess the magnitude of current and future space shortages. Using each department's footprint, a comparison is made between the current space allocation, the current space need (based on existing services, workload, equipment, staffing, and so on), and the future space need (based on program growth, new services, and anticipated operational and technology changes). The resulting preliminary space projections are used to develop facility reconfiguration options, site plans, and department block diagrams as part of the facility master plan. The planning horizon should correspond to the workload forecasts discussed in chapter 3. For the purposes of facility master planning, the space requirements of individual departments are estimated in the aggregate department gross square feet (DGSF), which differs from the detailed, room-by-room space programming in net square feet (NSF) as described in chapter 8. Detailed, room-by-room space programming is generally undertaken after specific projects have been defined as an outcome of the facility master plan.

Its approach to preliminary space planning depends on the organization's objectives, immediate issues, and corporate culture. The broad-brush approach is used to assess the overall scope of space deficiencies. Detailed, room-by-room space programming is not routinely performed at the facility master planning stage because it entails a tremendous amount of staff time and energy that is not appropriate for all departments, particularly those whose facilities are not an issue and whose status quo is assumed for the near future. In some cases, a more focused approach may be appropriate for one or more departments or service lines, and hospital leaders may fast track the detailed space programming process during facility master planning. Examples may include situations in which a competitive threat requires a shortened planning or design schedule, when code noncompliances must be rectified immediately, or when major pieces of equipment require urgent replacement. In these cases, a decision may be made to overlap the more detailed operational and space programming process for selected departments with the less detailed space planning assessment for all other departments during the facility master planning phase.

## TOOLS AND TECHNIQUES

At the onset of the facility master planning process, a preliminary list of all nursing units, departments, and functional areas should be assembled that corresponds to the institution's formal organizational structure or cost center listing. Specific tools and techniques are discussed in the following section.

### Focused Data Collection, Interviewing, and Surveying

Many facility planning consultants use standardized questionnaires to collect baseline data from department managers and medical directors. One questionnaire is typically used for nursing units (focused on licensed beds), another for clinical services where patients are treated in the department (focused on workload data and equipment), and another for all other support services that do not provide direct patient care (focused on staffing and processes). Baseline data are collected regarding the current scope of services, staffing and scheduling patterns, major equipment units, and workload. Surveys also solicit the perceptions of the department manager or medical director regarding current space deficiencies; workload trends; equipment suitability; and other anticipated changes in services, patient mix, processes, and technology. Focused interviews may then be conducted to assess the ability of the department or service line to accommodate the workload forecasts and operational and technological changes identified by the planning team, as described in chapters 3 and 4. A survey of the department's current space by an outside consultant or third party provides an objective assessment of the adequacy of current space allocation, quality of the space, equipment and procedure room use, and other facility planning issues.

## Using Benchmarks, Rules of Thumb, and Best Practices

Healthcare leaders frequently seek out industry benchmarks, rules of thumb, and best practices at other organizations around the country for validation. The healthcare sector uses different types of benchmarks, including those for assessing market demand (admissions per 1,000 population), financial performance (average cost per adjusted discharge), and labor productivity (full-time equivalents per occupied bed). For facility planning purposes, the most common types of benchmarks are those used to assess the following:

- Ability of the facilities to accommodate the current workload, such as the annual workload per treatment space
- Adequacy of overall space in a department to support the number of treatment spaces, such as the total DGSF per procedure room
- Space productivity, such as the annual procedures per DGSF
- Space efficiency, such as net-to-gross space ratios

Some examples of how benchmarks may be used to develop preliminary space estimates include the following (Hayward 2015):

- A surgery suite with 65 percent outpatient cases has 12 operating rooms (ORs) but accommodates only 9,600 annual cases (800 annual cases per OR); using a benchmark of 1,000 annual cases per OR, it would not need any additional ORs to accommodate the five-year growth projection of 12,000 annual cases.

◆ A dedicated outpatient surgery suite with six ORs currently has 15,000 DGSF (2,500 DGSF per OR), which is inadequate; using a benchmark of 3,000 DGSF per OR, hospital leadership determines that it requires 18,000 DGSF (an additional 3,000 DGSF).

Information regarding best practices in the healthcare sector, where the cost-effectiveness and improved quality outcomes have been substantiated relative to different operational models, can be found in many online sources.

## Incremental Need Approach

At this stage of the space planning process, common practice is to use an *incremental need approach* (as opposed to the *zero-based budget approach* employed during the detailed functional and space programming process). With the incremental need approach, space is added or subtracted from the current space allocation to reflect specific space deficiencies and surpluses in an individual department. For example, if a respiratory therapy department is currently assigned 4,300 DGSF and has two vacant offices, then planners can subtract approximately 300 DGSF from the current space allocation to arrive at the current space need of 4,000 DGSF. If at the same time this department has no temporary storage space for equipment that has been cleaned and is being held for disposition, then an estimated 100 DGSF would be added back into the current space allocation, resulting in a revised current space need of 4,100 DGSF.

These simple calculations are sufficient for use in preliminary space planning, where the goal is to understand the magnitude of the space deficiencies by major functional category of space. The subsequent development of a detailed, room-by-room space program may result in a slightly smaller or larger space estimate for an individual department.

## Scenario Analysis and Modeling

The effect of alternate workload and service configuration scenarios on space need is frequently predicted by developing appropriate assumptions and creating a computerized model or simple spreadsheet. For example, neonatal intensive care units (NICUs) are increasingly designed using either the single-family room (SFR) concept, semiprivate rooms to accommodate two infants, or a combination of both. Open-bay designs are primarily deployed where the constraints of existing space do not permit the other two options. To compare the space requirements of the SFR, semiprivate room, and open-bay facility configuration concepts, a space planning model was developed using common support-space assumptions while varying the patient care space. The total DGSF per bed for different sizes of NICUs was also evaluated. As shown in exhibit 5.1, for a smaller NICU with 12 beds, the semiprivate room and open-bay designs require about the same DGSF and the SFR unit requires about 7 percent more space. As the number of total beds increases, the differential between the SFR and open-bay concepts narrows. For a 24-bed NICU, the SFR layout requires 8 percent more space than semiprivate rooms do and only 5 percent more space than the open bays. The SFR concept requires 9 percent more space than the semiprivate room and 4 percent more space than the open-bay concept for a 36-bed NICU.

Guidelines for the minimum clear floor area required for each open bay have increased substantially in the past decade, which reduces the variance between the DGSF per bed in the open-bay design when compared with the SFR and semiprivate room options. Also, in this analysis, the open-bay concept provides additional sleeping rooms because recumbent sleeping facilities for parents are not bedside, as in the SFRs and semiprivate rooms.

When the DGSF per bed is reviewed in this example, the economies of scale of a larger unit far outweigh differences in facility configuration concept. NICUs with only SFRs range from 544 DGSF per bed for a 12-bed unit and decrease to 465 DGSF per bed for a 36-bed unit. Likewise, a unit with semiprivate rooms requires 507 DGSF per bed for a 12-bed unit, which decreases to 428 DGSF per bed for a 36-bed unit. The space required for a traditional open-bay NICU with 12 beds calculates to 509 DGSF per bed, which decreases to 445 DGSF per bed for a 36-bed unit. Healthcare leadership should also note that the net-to-gross conversion factor alone—assumed to be 1.50 in this example—represents one-third of the total DGSF per bed in such a way that a more efficient layout could mitigate differences between the facility configuration concept and the number of NICU beds.

It should be noted that as the number of NICU beds decreases further (i.e., fewer than 12 beds), the DGSF per bed increases substantially because of the minimum sizes required for support spaces. For example, a six-bed NICU, using the space planning model described in this analysis, would require more than 700 DGSF per bed.

## EVALUATING FACILITY CAPACITY

An analysis of facility capacity for clinical services involves identifying current workload volumes and major treatment spaces and then applying industry benchmarks

# Exhibit 5.1 Modeling the Space for Different Sizes and Configurations of NICUs

| | 12-Bed NICU | | | 24-Bed NICU | | | 36-Bed NICU | | |
|---|---|---|---|---|---|---|---|---|---|
| | Single-Family Rooms | Semiprivate Rooms | Open Bays | Single-Family Rooms | Semiprivate Rooms | Open Bays | Single-Family Rooms | Semiprivate Rooms | Open Bays |
| **Number of beds in:** | | | | | | | | | |
| Single-family rooms | 12 | — | — | 24 | — | — | 36 | — | — |
| Semiprivate rooms | — | 12 | — | — | 24 | — | — | 36 | — |
| Open bays | — | — | 12 | — | — | 24 | — | — | 36 |
| Total beds | 12 | 12 | 12 | 24 | 24 | 24 | 36 | 36 | 36 |
| **Net square feet (NSF):** | | | | | | | | | |
| Patient care (bed) space | 2,080 | 1,775 | 1,625 | 4,035 | 3,425 | 3,050 | 6,045 | 5,145 | 4,570 |
| Pod support space | — | — | — | 720 | 720 | 790 | 1,080 | 1,080 | 1,190 |
| Clinical support space | 755 | 755 | 755 | 910 | 910 | 910 | 1,010 | 1,010 | 1,010 |
| Staff support space | 695 | 695 | 695 | 1,200 | 1,200 | 1,200 | 1,475 | 1,475 | 1,475 |
| Family support space | 815 | 815 | 995 | 1,225 | 1,225 | 1,760 | 1,550 | 1,550 | 2,450 |
| Total NSF | 4,345 | 4,040 | 4,070 | 8,090 | 7,480 | 7,710 | 11,160 | 10,260 | 10,695 |
| Circulation space | 2,185 | 2,040 | 2,040 | 4,080 | 3,790 | 3,890 | 5,580 | 5,130 | 5,325 |
| Department gross square feet (DGSF) | 6,530 | 6,080 | 6,110 | 12,170 | 11,270 | 11,600 | 16,740 | 15,390 | 16,020 |
| DGSF per bed | 544 | 507 | 509 | 507 | 470 | 483 | 465 | 428 | 445 |

and rules of thumb. Evaluating the capacity of inpatient nursing units, however, is much more complicated if the organization was originally designed with a large number of multiple-bed patient rooms or has taken beds out of service at various points in time.

Even with adequate facility capacity, many healthcare organizations are limited in their weekly hours of operation because of the availability of physician, technical, and support staff. Shortages might result from scheduling difficulties, a tight job market, or regulatory and union issues with cross-training staff, for example. This scarcity is also true for inpatient nursing units—such as ICUs—where beds may be closed because of the inability to recruit nurses to staff them.

## Bed Capacity

Any capacity assessment should begin with an inventory and analysis of the inpatient nursing units, as described in chapter 2 and shown in exhibit 5.2. Inpatient nursing units are modular in design and consist of a number of patient rooms that typically share centralized support and administrative space. They vary in the number and type of patient rooms (private vs. multibed), the configuration of the contiguous toilet and bathing facilities, and the total DGSF used to support the specific number of beds.

As mentioned in chapter 2, the design capacity should be identified on the basis of physical inspection of the unit and current architectural drawings. Historically, as the census declined, many organizations began taking beds out of service and typically redeployed selected patient rooms on each unit to accommodate increasing equipment storage needs, new ancillary and clinical staff, or point-of-care services. In some cases, headwalls were removed and toilet and bathing facilities reconfigured; in other cases, these features were preserved so that the rooms could be redeployed with minimal cost as demand changed. The design capacity refers to the total number of beds that could be redeployed for patient care with minimal renovation—for example, patient rooms temporarily used as offices or storage rooms with the headwalls and utilities still intact.

Exhibit 5.2 shows a breakdown of a hospital with 290 total beds, including the following details:

- The nursing units located in the newer east wing provide generously sized private patient rooms with contemporary toilet and bathing facilities and appropriate support space.
- The nursing units located in the north wing have a sufficient number of private rooms (79 percent) and an appropriate amount of space per

bed (507 DGSF). Although six of the beds on each unit are located in semiprivate rooms, with 25 patient rooms and 28 beds on each unit, the semiprivate rooms would not need to be occupied by more than one patient until the census exceeds about 90 percent.

- The older units in the south wing have few private rooms and an inadequate amount of space to support the staffed beds (283 to 354 DGSF per bed).
- The rehabilitation unit (4-South Wing) is particularly problematic, with only 283 DGSF per bed and no private rooms. Rehabilitation units with an extended length of stay generally require more DGSF per bed than an acute care nursing unit to provide central dining, therapy, and family and visitor space; with all beds in semiprivate rooms, high occupancy rates are unlikely.
- Even though the hospital possesses design capacity for an additional 11 beds in the south wing, deployment of former patient rooms is unlikely, given that the support space is already insufficient for the beds currently staffed.
- Although the south wing is severely lacking in private patient rooms, simply converting the semiprivate rooms to private rooms would not be an option because it would reduce the unit sizes in such a way that efficient staffing patterns would not be possible—for example, a 14-bed unit.
- Compared with the medical/surgical intensive care unit (MSICU), the cardiothoracic intensive care unit (CICU) is severely undersized (364 versus 692 DGSF per bed); one of the original ten patient rooms in the CICU has already been redeployed for equipment storage.
- The mother–baby unit was originally designed with all semiprivate rooms, but 12 of the original semiprivates are used as privates because of declining census; support space is adequate for the 20 beds currently staffed.
- The pediatric unit staffs all of the original semiprivate rooms as single-bed rooms, but because of the continued low census and the shift to same-day and outpatient settings, the nine rooms are often used as an overflow for adult same-day and observation patients.

Although not shown in exhibit 5.2, comparison of the NSF of the patient rooms (inside wall-to-wall dimension, excluding the toilet and bathing facilities and the access alcove) is also useful if a variety of nursing units had been constructed or upgraded at different points in time. A review of the NSF of a typical private and semiprivate patient room on each nursing unit indicates whether an inadequate DGSF per bed ratio is a result of minimally sized patient rooms or a lack of support space, or both. Any code-compliance issues with either the size of the patient rooms or the size and access to the contiguous patient toilet and bathing facilities should also be identified.

# Exhibit 5.2 Example: Nursing Unit Capacity Analysis

| Service | Capacity | Staffed Beds | | Staffed Beds in | | | Space | |
|---|---|---|---|---|---|---|---|---|
| | Total Beds | Beds | Rooms | Private Rooms | Double Rooms | Private Beds (%) | DGSF | DGSF/Bed |
| *General medical/surgical units* | | | | | | | | |
| 3-East Wing (medical/surgical) | 36 | 36 | 36 | 36 | — | 100 | 24,300 | 675 |
| 4-East Wing (cardiovascular) | 36 | 36 | 36 | 36 | — | 100 | 24,300 | 675 |
| 2-North Wing (medical/surgical) | 28 | 28 | 25 | 22 | 6 | 79 | 14,200 | 507 |
| 3-North Wing (medical/surgical) | 28 | 28 | 25 | 22 | 6 | 79 | 14,200 | 507 |
| 2-South Wing (medical/surgical) | 28 | 24 | 14 | 4 | 20 | 17 | 8,500 | 354 |
| 3-South Wing (ortho/neuro/urology) | 30 | 25 | 15 | 5 | 20 | 20 | 8,760 | 350 |
| 4-South Wing (rehabilitation) | 32 | 30 | 15 | — | 30 | 0 | 8,490 | 283 |
| **Subtotal (general medical/surgical)** | 218 | 207 | 166 | 125 | 82 | 60 | 102,750 | 496 |
| *Critical care units* | | | | | | | | |
| 1-MSICU (medical/surgical intensive care unit) | 12 | 12 | 12 | 12 | — | 100 | 8,300 | 692 |
| 1-CICU (cardiothoracic intensive care unit) | 10 | 9 | 9 | 9 | — | 100 | 3,280 | 364 |
| **Subtotal (critical care)** | 22 | 21 | 21 | 21 | — | 100 | 11,580 | 551 |
| **Subtotal (medical/surgical)** | 240 | 228 | 187 | 146 | 82 | 64 | 114,330 | 501 |
| *Maternal/child units* | | | | | | | | |
| 3-East (mother–baby unit) | 32 | 20 | 16 | 12 | 8 | 60 | 9,960 | 498 |
| 3-West (pediatrics/overflow adult) | 18 | 9 | 9 | 9 | 9 | 100 | 6,500 | 722 |
| **Subtotal (maternal/child)** | 50 | 29 | 25 | 21 | 17 | 72 | 16,460 | 568 |
| **Total** | 290 | 257 | 212 | 167 | 99 | 65 | 130,790 | 509 |

## Capacity of Major Clinical Services

Healthcare organizations vary to a surprising degree in the number of expensive procedure rooms and equipment units that they use to accommodate similar numbers of annual procedures. This variation is why it is important to look at the current capacity of specific clinical services prior to expanding the number of procedure rooms and related support space, particularly those services that use expensive equipment and require uniquely designed procedure rooms. Key questions to ask prior to committing significant dollars to expanding or upgrading a department include the following:

- Is the current equipment state of the art? Would newer, upgraded equipment improve throughput and thus eliminate the need for additional procedure rooms? Can the current procedure rooms accommodate new, upgraded equipment, considering size and dimensions, ceiling height, floor loading capacity, and power and telecommunications requirements?
- Could the daily and weekly hours of operation be extended to allow more procedures to be performed per week with the existing or upgraded equipment, such as staffing the department during evening or weekend hours?
- Even if the current number of procedure rooms is sufficient, is support space adequate to allow the department to function efficiently and to meet customer service needs, including staff work areas; supply storage; and patient waiting, reception, preparation, and recovery space?
- Would relocating the department to an alternate location facilitate the sharing of staff, enhance customer convenience, or allow procedure rooms or support space to be shared with another department or service?
- Would a newly configured or relocated department reduce staffing costs, increase workloads and corresponding revenue, or provide other quantitative benefits that would balance the initial capital cost of equipment acquisition and facility renovation or construction?

Exhibit 5.3 summarizes general capacity benchmarks for key diagnostic and treatment services, assuming target procedure room turnaround times and moderate technology implementation. The exhibit then identifies the optimal annual number of procedures that a single piece of equipment or procedure room can accommodate. The annual capacity is determined by first identifying the number of procedures or visits that can optimally be scheduled in an hour, as well as the number of hours per day that the department will be staffed, and then by assuming

**Exhibit 5.3 Capacity Benchmarks for Major Diagnostic Treatment Services**

| Service/Workload Unit | Category | Average Annual Workload per Treatment Space | Average DGSF per Treatment Space |
|---|---|---|---|
| Emergency visits | ED treatment | 1,200–1,600 | 550–650 |
| | Fast-track treatment | 1,800–2,400 | 400–450 |
| Surgery cases | Inpatients primarily (< 35% outpatients) | 700–800 | 2,800–3,000 |
| | Inpatient–outpatient mix (50% outpatients) | 800–900 | 3,000–3,500 |
| | Inpatient–outpatient mix (> 65% outpatients) | 900–1,000 | 3,200–3,500 |
| | Outpatient suite | 1,250–1,500 | 3,000–3,500 |
| Endoscopy procedures | Small suite (2–3 procedure rooms) | 1,250–1,500 | 1,500–2,000 |
| | Medium suite (3–4 procedure rooms) | 1,250–2,000+ | 1,250–1,500 |
| | Large suite (5–6 procedure rooms) | 1,500–2,000+ | 1,000–1,250 |
| Obstetrics births | LDRP exclusively | 100–200 | 800–1,000 |
| | LDR primarily | 300–400 | |
| Imaging procedures | General radiography/fluoroscopy | 5,000–6,000 | 800–1,000 |
| | Computed tomography (CT) | 8,000–10,000 | 1,200–1,500 |
| | Magnetic resonance imaging (MRI) | 4,000–6,000 | 1,400–1,700 |
| | Nuclear medicine | 1,200–2,000 | 1,200–1,600 |
| | Ultrasound | 2,000–2,500 | 600–700 |
| | Interventional imaging | 900–1,800 | 2,000–2,400 |
| Radiation oncology visits | First linear accelerator/gamma knife treatment room | 6,500+ | 7,000–8,000 |
| | Per additional treatment room | | 5,000–6,000 |
| Medical oncology visits | Chemotherapy/infusion | 500–1,500 | 250–350 |
| Physician office visits | Private physician office | 2,400–4,500 | 400–450 |
| | Faculty/resident clinic | 1,000–2,000 | 450–600 |

*Source:* Adapted from Hayward (2015).

50 weeks per year of operation (allowing for about ten holidays). Some factors that influence procedure room turnaround time include the following:

- *Technology.* With a traditional, single-slice computed tomography (CT) scanner, patients were scheduled every 30 minutes so that each procedure room could accommodate 16 patient studies or procedures per day based on an eight-hour day. The newer scanners can acquire multiple images per second, resulting in an average procedure time of less than ten minutes. This efficiency allows four patients to be scheduled per hour, or twice the number as with the older unit.
- *Patient mix and scheduling patterns.* Physician practice space and clinics will have varying use of their exam rooms depending on the type of patients being seen (e.g., dermatology, general surgery, oncology, and pediatrics), teaching obligations, and scheduling patterns such as evening and weekend sessions.
- *Responsiveness of support services.* The time required to prepare a surgical OR for the next case (OR turnover time) has a significant impact on the daily number of cases that can be accommodated in a single OR.
- *Responsiveness of other hospital departments.* The turnaround of emergency department (ED) exam and treatment cubicles is greatly influenced by the responsiveness of the central laboratory and imaging departments if point-of-care services are not available; a shortage of inpatient beds can cause patients, who need to be admitted, to back up in the ED. The responsiveness of consulting physicians also affects patient throughput.

## Physician Practice Space and Outpatient Clinics

Physician practice space was traditionally planned assuming two exam rooms and an office for each physician. The space was dedicated for use by a specific physician, regardless of the hours per week he was present. Because of the competing responsibilities of most physicians, exam rooms were typically underused, especially on Monday mornings and Fridays, with peak demand midweek. The variance between peak-volume and low-volume days is even more pronounced in academic medical centers, where medical faculty also have teaching and research responsibilities that further reduce (and affect the scheduling of) their time in outpatient clinics.

The space needed for physician practices and outpatient clinics is usually based on the anticipated schedule and staffing patterns. Planners typically provide two exam rooms per provider, although high-volume, quick-turnaround specialties—such as dermatology and orthopedics—may effectively use three exam rooms per provider. However, the weekly number of visits per exam room should also be calculated to identify whether exam rooms are being fully used. For example, 400 visits per week (Monday through Friday, eight hours per day) with 24 exam rooms result in an average of 3.3 visits per exam room per day. If patients are typically scheduled two per hour in a particular clinic, an occupancy rate of only 21 percent results. In this case, alteration of the planned scheduling pattern should be considered so that fewer half-day clinic sessions per week are scheduled, resulting in the potential reassignment of the exam rooms to another provider team during other times of the week.

Providers typically schedule a range of one to four patients per hour. This variation depends on the physician's specialty and the proportion of new patient visits to return or follow-up visits, which affects the length of time that the patient spends in the exam room. I generally use an exam room occupancy rate of 90 percent for private practitioners who do not have a high number of no-show patients. Teaching clinics, where care is provided primarily by residents supervised by academic physicians (who, when considered together, spend longer times with patients) and where there is a large number of no-shows, typically see the fewest number of patients per exam room per day. In this case, I would use an exam room occupancy rate of 70 percent for planning purposes.

Well-planned physician practice space and outpatient clinics provide sufficient intrinsic flexibility to accommodate sizable deviations from workload forecasts. This adaptability is accomplished by creating spaces that can be used interchangeably for various types of visits; understanding the relationships among workload, service times, and staffing to respond to unexpected surges in workload; and accommodating a wide range of patient visits in a single flexible exam or treatment space. For example, if ten patients are typically seen per exam room per day, extending the daily schedule to 7 pm allows the same space to accommodate a 25 percent increase in annual workload. Moreover, using the exam rooms to see patients for eight hours on Saturday increases the weekly capacity by another 20 percent (48 hours per week versus 40 hours).

## UNDERSTANDING YOUR OUTPATIENT POPULATION

The explosive growth in outpatient care in the 1980s, 1990s, and early 2000s, coupled with an intense focus on patient convenience, led to a proliferation of dedicated and freestanding outpatient facilities on and off campus. Unfortunately, it has been my observation that some of these new outpatient facilities increased operational costs but brought in little incremental revenue to support the redundant staff, equipment, and space. As noted in chapter 1, the healthcare industry has recently experienced a reverse migration of sorts. Hospitals are aggressively acquiring private physician practices and independent ambulatory surgery and diagnostic centers and converting them to hospital outpatient departments to optimize reimbursement for hospitals and lessen the risk for the existing owners. Of course, this trend can reverse at any point depending on reimbursement and other financial incentives.

A healthcare organization should understand its current outpatient population before embarking on facility master planning. This understanding requires at least an initial analysis of how many and what types of outpatients come to the hospital campus on a typical day, in addition to their specific destinations; an example of this type of analysis is shown in exhibit 5.4. Typical daily outpatient visits can be estimated by dividing the annual workload by the annual days of operation of the specific service and then applying a factor to account for scheduling variations throughout the week and by shift, as applicable. For example, you can generally assume that 10–20 percent more patients will visit the campus on the peak weekday than on the average. In the case of the ED, you can assume that 50 percent of the estimated daily emergency visits will occur on the busiest shift.

**Exhibit 5.4 Example: Typical Daily Outpatient Visits by Service and Destination—Hospital-Sponsored Only (n = 1,423)**

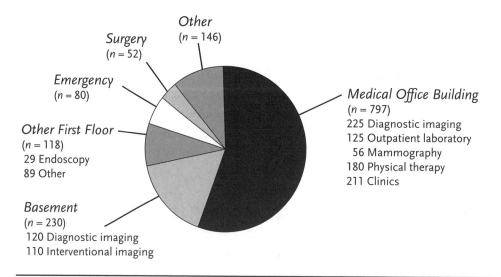

Surgery
(n = 52)

Other
(n = 146)

Emergency
(n = 80)

Other First Floor
(n = 118)
29 Endoscopy
89 Other

Basement
(n = 230)
120 Diagnostic imaging
110 Interventional imaging

Medical Office Building
(n = 797)
225 Diagnostic imaging
125 Outpatient laboratory
 56 Mammography
180 Physical therapy
211 Clinics

# BENCHMARKING YOUR CURRENT FUNCTIONAL LAYOUT AGAINST TEN FACILITY CONFIGURATION PRINCIPLES

Whether expanding or reconfiguring an existing campus or planning an entirely new healthcare campus, key questions for hospital planners should include the following:

- How well do we orient our customers as they arrive on the campus and circulate through the facilities?
- Are the facilities configured to use staff efficiently and allow the sharing of valuable space and expensive equipment?
- Is the space organized and configured to provide the most cost-effective setting for any given function?

You can perform a mini-assessment of the current functional layout of your facilities and identify potential issues by comparing your current site and facilities to the following ten optimal configuration principles:

1.  *Separate key types of campus traffic.* Site access points should be clearly marked with directional signage to relevant parking lots and easily identifiable building entrance points for emergency traffic, service traffic, and public and visitor traffic heading for patient intake and admission, medical office buildings, or various outpatient services. External signage should be reviewed with the fresh eyes of someone who is unfamiliar with the specific campus to identify issues relative to misleading, incomprehensible, or inconsistent destination names and directional signs that are unreadable or absent.

2.  *Clearly define the front door.* Just as most shopping centers are designed with a single prominent entrance to assist first-time customers who are unfamiliar with the overall layout and require orientation, healthcare centers should generally have a clearly defined main entrance or "front door" supplemented by ancillary entrances that patients will be encouraged to use on subsequent visits (leading directly to their service destination). Ideally, with a well-designed patient information and communication system, patients should be provided with a campus map and directions to their destination prior to their arrival.

3.  *Coordinate and colocate customer intake and access services.* A single, one-stop shopping location, or customer service center, should be provided immediately inside the main entrance. Services should include patient and visitor reception; information dissemination; admitting, registration, and

insurance verification; family support services; and amenities. From this central hub, other patient and visitor services can be coordinated.

4. *Optimize the use of prime real estate.* Services that involve customer interaction and face-to-face contact should be concentrated on the grade-level floor adjacent to the front door or major outpatient entrances. The use of this prime real estate for administrative offices and other support services that could be located remotely should be discouraged.

5. *Minimize the total number of outpatient destinations.* Related clinical services should be grouped around a centralized reception and intake area or "destination" marked with clear and consistent directional signage. For example, patients can be directed to the Diagnostic Center reception and waiting area from which they are escorted to the point of care—radiology, nuclear medicine, CT, magnetic resonance imaging (MRI), for example— when the staff members and procedure room are available. Diagramming the current number of possible outpatient destinations and the routes required to reach them also identifies inconvenient service locations and wayfinding issues.

6. *Position diagnostic and treatment services for changing technology and future operational flexibility* by colocating services with similar facility needs such as routine, quick-turnaround procedures (e.g., phlebotomy and simple X-rays); specialty imaging; interventional services; and surgery and same-day medical procedures.

7. *Minimize inpatient transfers* by providing private patient rooms (to the extent possible), organizing inpatient nursing units by specialty rather than acuity (depending on volumes), and implementing the acuity adaptable patient room concept (where possible).

8. *Unbundle high-volume, recurring outpatient services to an off-site location.* If contiguous parking and convenient access cannot be achieved on the main campus, high-volume, recurring outpatient services should be relocated off-site; examples include outpatient physical therapy, outpatient behavioral health, intravenous or infusion therapy, and outpatient dialysis.

9. *Unbundle building support services.* Space for building support services should be located in inexpensive construction (on- or off-site), though it should still facilitate efficient material distribution to key users such as inpatient nursing units or the surgery suite.

10. *Provide flexible, generic administrative office space.* Larger office suites should be planned (on- or off-site) in lieu of smaller pockets of offices throughout the hospital campus. Flexible, generic office space should be planned to accommodate department staff members who do not require face-to-face

contact with customers so that offices and workstations can be reassigned periodically as programs and staffing levels change.

## SUMMARIZING SPACE REQUIREMENTS

Using each department's footprint, a comparison should be made between the current space allocation, the current space need (based on current services, workload, and resources), and the future space need (based on program growth, new services, and anticipated operational and technological changes). Space should be organized and subtotaled by the major functional categories discussed in chapter 2. The planning horizon should correspond to the workload forecasts (typically five years), and multiple scenarios may be modeled to reflect varied assumptions regarding bed need and ancillary workloads. In addition, space efficiencies that could be achieved by consolidating departments either on-site or off-site should be identified. The future space projections should be based on a foundation of supporting data and an objective assessment of actual need rather than solely on department or service line manager perceptions.

## SUMMARIZING KEY FACILITY ISSUES AND ESTABLISHING PRIORITIES

Because it may not be practical (or feasible) to solve all facility problems in a given planning horizon, the importance of individual problems must be evaluated in relation to one another. To make capital investment decisions during the facility master planning process, an organization must be able to understand the magnitude and the relative urgency of facility problems. Ideally, all departments and services should be evaluated against a common set of criteria to ensure that investments are not just directed toward the "squeaky wheel" and to identify issues that have not yet been raised. These criteria may range from operational concerns to issues with a department's location and internal layout, along with specific physical plant issues. Evaluation criteria can be separated into overall facility planning issues and specific space deficiencies.

Facility planning issues for most hospital services or departments include the following:

◆ *Workload capacity.* The current facilities cannot accommodate recent workload growth, or surplus capacity exists.

- *Operational processes.* Inappropriate policies or difficulties with staff recruiting prevent efficient scheduling or limit the use of procedure rooms.
- *Functional layout.* The internal department layout impedes smooth and efficient workflow.
- *Location and linkages.* The space and functional layout of the department may be adequate, but the location is remote from related patient and support services.
- *Equipment and technology.* The medical equipment is outdated or unreliable, or obsolete information technology systems are still employed.
- *Image and interior decor.* The furnishings are worn out and the interior decor is outdated.
- *Physical plant or environment.* The facility experiences issues related to temperature control, electrical shortages, plumbing leaks, vibrations, and so on.
- *Codes or regulations.* Code noncompliances have been cited by regulatory agencies, and a plan for rectification must be developed.

Each of the potential issues described on this list has different cost and timing implications for the organization.

Specific space issues can be categorized according to the type of space that is deficient:

- *Patient care and treatment space*, including prep, exam and consultation, procedure, and recovery space as well as inpatient rooms—all necessary to provide an appropriate work environment for clinicians; accommodate new equipment and technology; and ensure patient safety, privacy, and comfort
- *Clinical support space*, such as clean and soiled workrooms, medication rooms, and equipment storage space
- *Staff support space*, such as staff offices, workstations, conference rooms, lounges, and toilet facilities
- *Customer intake space and amenities*, including reception, registration, waiting areas, and other amenities (e.g., toilet facilities, food service)

Additional issues related to inpatient nursing units include a lack of private patient rooms, the size of the patient room, inadequate toilet and bathing facilities, and accommodations for special patient populations (e.g., handicapped, bariatric, geriatric, and infectious disease patients).

The types of facility issues and space deficiencies have different implications as well. Inappropriately sized and configured treatment areas with outdated equipment and technology may affect the quality of care and increase medical errors, while inadequate staff workstations may negatively affect staff recruiting and retention. The lack of patient and visitor support space, amenities, and outdated interior decor and furnishings may promote a negative first impression among the organization's customers and defeat efforts to expand market share and increase workload volumes.

## USING MATRICES

As shown in exhibit 5.5, facility planners may use a matrix format during the facility master planning process to present key facility issues in a concise manner, identifying common problems and facilitating priority setting.

As each department is evaluated against a common set of criteria, major and minor issues may be further delineated. Finally, each department should be prioritized according to a scale that is relevant to the specific organization. For example, departments may be assigned one of the following priorities:

- *High priority* requires that a solution be developed and implemented within two years. However, in the case of new construction, a high-priority project may take five years or more for completion, so that the planning will need to start immediately.
- *Medium priority* requires that a solution be developed and implemented in two to five years.
- *Low priority* assumes the status quo is adequate or that a solution does not need to be developed or implemented within a five-year planning horizon.

The primary goal of this type of analysis is to separate the departments and service lines with more critical facility issues from those that require little attention over a specific period. This delineation allows the facility planning effort to proceed efficiently in a logical, focused manner. Facility planners should note, however, that a department with no facility issues may still need to be relocated or reconfigured to allow another department's high-priority issues to be resolved.

As discussed in chapter 6, department staff and physicians may feel that their facilities are inadequate for reasons ranging from equipment and technology deficiencies to outdated furnishings to actual code noncompliances. In many cases, the solution is not necessarily an updated or expanded facility. Separating staff perceptions from actual facility needs is critical to a successful facility master planning process.

# Exhibit 5.5 Example: Summarizing Key Facility Issues Using Matrices

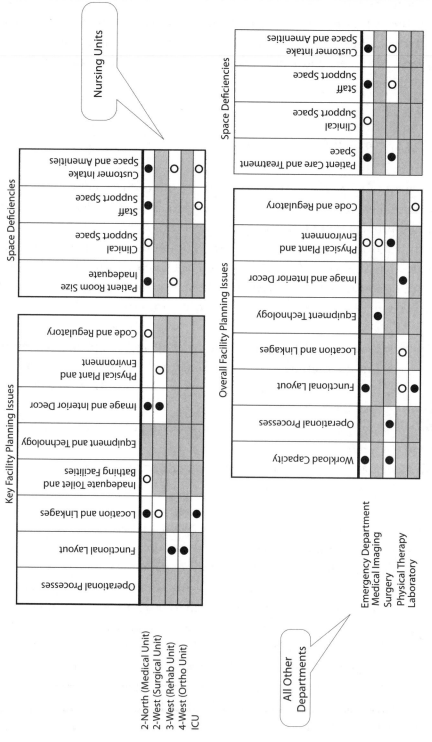

## SPECIFIC ISSUES ASSOCIATED WITH ELIMINATING SURPLUS CAPACITY

Healthcare organizations spent much effort in the past to eliminate surplus capacity in response to declining inpatient admissions and length of stay, overbuilt outpatient facilities, shrinking hospital-based diagnostic and treatment departments, and oversized building support space (such as the laundry, warehouse, and kitchen) originally designed for a much larger hospital chassis at a time when hospitals provided all services on-site. In 2013, the number of hospitals and hospital beds involved in mergers reached a five-year high (American Hospital Association and Avalere Health 2014). One of the many challenges that newly merged multihospital healthcare systems face is eliminating redundant services and surplus capacity. The realignment of services and reallocation of resources among multiple campuses require a unique strategic, operations improvement, and facility planning process. Alternate ways of allocating resources should be thoroughly evaluated and the impact on operational costs fully understood prior to spending money on bricks and mortar. Multihospital healthcare systems also need to understand the market and patient population served at each of the individual hospital campuses. A different facility planning approach is required when two or more campuses, or sites, share the same market than when they have distinctly separate markets. Planning at the service line level is also required because some service lines may share the same market and others may not. For example, consolidating two obstetrics programs at a single location could negatively affect the health system's market share for this service line if the new location is deemed inconvenient for the referring physicians and patients.

Although hospital leadership may find many opportunities to eliminate surplus capacity, the following key areas represent the most significant opportunities.

### Eliminating Empty Beds

Although consolidating occupied beds into larger nursing units and closing complete floors or converting them to an alternate use can have some impact on operational costs, the real cost savings occur when entire hospitals are closed. The dramatic reduction in inpatient length of stay in the past has not been because all the patients who traditionally occupied acute care beds were being treated in freestanding outpatient facilities or were simply being discharged from the hospital and sent home sooner. Same-day procedures or short stays have increased, particularly in the case of Medicare patients who may be assigned observation status, even though they are held in the hospital overnight. This growing group of acute ambu-latory (short-stay) patients are often sicker and less ambulatory than traditional outpatients. Conversion of some surplus acute care bed capacity for observation units or post-acute services may be an option depending on the overall condition of the infrastructure and code compliance of the facility.

## Integrating and Restructuring Clinical Services

Historically, hospitals have had a reputation for being inefficient and compartmen-talized, with high overhead and inflexible full-time employees. Departmental turf wars for real estate, resources, and supplies are still common. These problems only get worse when two hospitals try to merge their operations. However, the rationale for a merger between two or more hospitals is often stated as something such as this: "The new healthcare environment demands a leaner, downsized, more nimble, bottom line–oriented business enterprise." Opportunities to reduce surplus capac-ity through clinical service integration include the following:

- Consolidating expensive diagnostic and treatment services
- Identifying the lowest-cost and most appropriate setting to deliver outpatient care—episodic, acute, routine, and chronic or recurring care
- Evaluating extended hours of operation in lieu of equipment acquisition and more space to further improve use of resources
- Investigating the center of excellence or "institute" concept as an alternative to traditional organizational models
- Restructuring routine, high-volume, quick-turnaround testing to improve patient access and to share staff and space

## Consolidating Physician Practices

As more physician practices become part of larger specialty groups, opportunities arise to reduce operating costs by sharing resources. Some possibilities include sharing reception and registration, waiting space, and other patient and staff amenities; sharing of support staff, thus reducing the need for offices and work-stations; and sharing specialized staff, expensive treatment and special procedure rooms, and diagnostic facilities. The number of exam rooms can also be reduced by improving their throughput; time sharing; and by planning more generic, flexible space.

## Reducing Building Support Space

Most of today's hospitals were designed with a chassis for a much larger number of inpatient beds than patients currently occupy. Space for support services is commonly located in the basement, or below grade. When two organizations merge, the surplus space further increases. Many multihospital systems have implemented the *mosaic approach* by designating certain campuses for consolidation of specific services, thus reducing their investment in duplicate and redundant resources. For example, a single kitchen may be located at one site (with the cook-chill system used to deliver food to the remaining sites) and a single warehouse located at another site from which supplies are distributed.

## Remembering that Nature Abhors a Vacuum

When there is ample surplus space, hospital departments tend to metastasize into the space available, whether or not all the space is needed. This leads to a lack of appreciation for space as an important asset, and it may result in an exaggerated space allocation when the department is relocated to leased space or an alternate facility and the incremental need approach is used to estimate the size of the new space.

## Separating Major Consolidation Issues from Nonissues

Paralysis often sets in when recently merged institutions begin consolidation planning. Assuming that market dynamics and demographics have been carefully considered, the key is to quickly separate actual facility consolidation issues from nonissues. Questions that should be initially addressed when considering the consolidation of one or more acute care hospitals at a single site include the following:

- Are there contemporary inpatient nursing units in a modern physical plant with code-compliant, appropriately sized patient rooms and adjoining toilet and bathing facilities? What percentage of the beds are in private patient rooms? How many total patient "rooms" are available? What amount of renovation or construction would be required to provide all private patient rooms?
- Are surgical operating rooms, including open-heart and hybrid rooms, updated and adequately sized? What is the capacity, considering extended hours of operation?

- Are there contemporary obstetrical labor and delivery facilities? What is the capacity assuming that a single-room maternity model may not be achievable?
- What are the size and number of specialty imaging procedure rooms for procedures such as CT, MRI, interventional radiology and cardiology, and radiation therapy? Is the technology state of the art?
- What is the customer's first impression of each facility? Are there convenient patient access, adequate parking, and a welcoming entrance lobby? Is the facility surrounded by green space, or is it a landlocked site with adversarial neighbors?
- Is there room on the site for building or parking expansion?
- What is the amount, proximity, and ownership of specialty physician offices on each site, particularly if one site will potentially be abandoned?

Less important issues are often given more attention than warranted include diagnostic and treatment services that do not involve large fixed equipment or require specific design requirements—for example, ultrasound and physical therapy—and any department whose space consists primarily of offices and workstations.


## Political, Emotional, and Regulatory Issues

Despite the high number of hospitals in the United States involved in mergers, acquisitions, or joint ventures since the mid-1990s, my experience with multihospital systems indicates that the urgency to eliminate surplus capacity and achieve the corresponding operational cost savings often coincides with points at which the health system runs out of cash and debt capacity.

Russ Coile (Coile and Hayward 1997) observes that "deeply entrenched economic interests and local politics are serious considerations which any healthcare executive must overcome when recommending consolidation or closure." He cites a number of political and emotional factors, including regulatory issues and the involvement of state attorneys general; community opposition and public relations problems; unions, displaced workers, and the economic impact on the community; and the effect on local philanthropy when a hospital is closed.

Abandoning facilities with new additions or recently renovated space creates unique emotional and political issues. Physician ownership of office space and diagnostic facilities on or near a hospital site to be abandoned further complicates the equation. The opportunities for cost savings, however, are tremendous. Funds used to support surplus capacity could be deployed for a long list of alternate purposes, including the eventual replacement of the core physical plant and technology of the surviving institutions. Unfortunately, funds spent on postponing the inevitable will not be available for investment in the future, and decisions to fund operating losses are rarely evaluated relative to the lost opportunity.

## REFERENCES

American Hospital Association and Avalere Health. 2014. *TrendWatch Chartbook 2014: Trends Affecting Hospitals and Health Systems*. Accessed January 13, 2016. www.aha.org/research/reports/tw/chartbook/2014/14chartbook.pdf.

Coile, R. C., Jr., and C. Hayward. 1997. "Excess Hospital Capacity: Recycling, Retrofitting (or Closure!): Alternatives for America's Excess Inpatient Beds." *Russ Coile's Health Trends* (10) 1: 3–8.

Hayward, C. 2015. *SpaceMed Guide: A Space Planning Guide for Healthcare Facilities*, 3rd ed. Ann Arbor, MI: HA Ventures.

# CHAPTER 6

# Reaching Consensus on a Long-Range Facility Investment Strategy

IN THE TRADITIONAL facility master planning process, space deficiencies and projections are often translated directly into facility options that are represented by architectural drawings. A preferred design solution is subsequently selected. Renovation or construction cost estimates and a phased construction schedule are developed, with individual projects identified for funding approval and staged implementation. As part of the implementation of the facility master plan, the design architect is then commissioned to provide more detailed architectural drawings and to prepare construction documents.

The problem with this approach is that alternative operational concepts are often evaluated (if evaluated at all) on the basis of an architectural rendering rather than sound business principles and consistency with specific strategic planning and operations improvement objectives. For example, in this phase, the architect may draw alternative surgery suite configurations—such as a combined inpatient and outpatient suite versus a separate outpatient surgery suite—when such a decision should have been made prior to the design process and should be based on an evaluation of case mix and workload volumes, operational costs, surgeon preferences, revenue generation, and customer access. This kind of facility master planning process, where the planning team jumps prematurely into design with the sole output being an architectural block drawing of planned future department locations and building projects, is no longer relevant given the dynamic nature of the healthcare sector. If market conditions change and workload projections do not come to fruition in such a way that one or more projects prove infeasible, or if department leadership changes, the entire plan is deemed outdated and then is shelved.

## WHY DEVELOP A LONG-RANGE FACILITY INVESTMENT STRATEGY?

The gap between the identification of facility deficiencies and future space needs and the search for subsequent architectural solutions should be bridged with a thorough evaluation of priorities and capital investment trade-offs. Consensus on the resulting long-range facility development strategy, or capital investment strategy, allows the planning team to begin a phased implementation of the facility master plan with confidence. It can readily alter its course as needed to reflect unanticipated changes in the market, reimbursement, regulations, and technology.

A long-range facility investment strategy essentially provides a road map to guide renovation and construction (and capital investment) over a defined planning horizon. It helps senior leadership to understand key facility issues and priorities facing the organization and to reach consensus on capital investment goals and objectives. It also aligns facility investments with the organization's strategic (market) plan, operations improvement initiatives, planned information technology (IT) investments (IT strategic plan), and financial resources. Documentation of an agreed-on facility investment strategy assists in the education of physicians, employees, and other stakeholders relative to long-range planning goals and priorities. Unlike the traditional facility master plan, adherence to defined strategies allows for a dynamic process that does not become obsolete if one or more individual projects are derailed.

## COMMON STRATEGIES DEVELOPED BY HEALTHCARE ORGANIZATIONS TODAY

From my experience, the most common facility investment strategies developed by healthcare organizations generally involve the following:

- Bed allocation and nursing unit reconfiguration
- Clinical services reconfiguration and upgrading
- Outpatient services configuration and provision of physician office space
- Building infrastructure upgrading and equipment acquisition or replacement
- Patient experience improvement

## Bed Allocation and Nursing Unit Reconfiguration

Today, much of the costly inpatient care in the United States is still delivered in facilities that were designed when cost-based reimbursement was the norm, nurses were easy to recruit, and the nurse-call system was considered high-tech. Inpatient care is often fragmented into small, specialized units organized by acuity level, with much of the care delivered by specialists from large, centralized ancillary departments. Simple patient care activities, such as a chest X-ray or a blood test, may require numerous steps and personnel, resulting in prolonged turnaround times, delayed decision making, extended lengths of stay, and ultimately increased costs. Along with a high number of semiprivate patient rooms, these characteristics result in frequent patient transfers that involve multiple departments and members of the staff throughout the organization. After being encouraged over the past two decades to reduce surplus inpatient bed capacity in response to declining admissions, use rates, and lengths of stay, some hospitals are struggling to accommodate growing inpatient volumes—particularly high-acuity patients.

Because of the large amount of space devoted to inpatient care in the typical hospital, with inpatient care representing a disproportionately large percentage of an organization's total costs, healthcare organizations with aging facilities need to develop a strategy for reconfiguring inefficient nursing units, updating outdated facilities, and in some cases expanding or replacing beds. A long-range facility reconfiguration plan should address inpatient nursing unit configuration by service line, acuity, and type of patient accommodation—private, semiprivate, short-stay, and observation—and should correspond to anticipated high bed and low bed scenarios. For healthcare organizations with inadequate accommodations for high-acuity patients, a large number of semiprivate rooms, and aging facilities, a phased plan for ongoing bed replacement is necessary. Potential bed expansion must also be addressed in growing markets with aging populations.

As discussed in chapter 3, identifying the range of beds that may be needed and then developing a flexible facility investment strategy that can be adjusted as certain benchmarks are achieved are important for facility planning purposes. Specific strategies may involve the following:

- Constructing additional new beds to meet the high bed scenario, or replacing some of the existing, outdated beds with new beds if the high bed scenario turns out to be overly aggressive
- Constructing larger acuity adaptable patient rooms that have the ability to accommodate acute or critical care patients as needed

- Redeploying existing patient rooms as either privates or semiprivates to offset inaccuracies in projecting future demand
- Developing an observation unit that is less expensive and quicker to construct than a traditional inpatient nursing unit to supplement inpatient bed need

## Clinical Services Reconfiguration and Upgrading

Healthcare organizations are reconfiguring and often realigning clinical services among multiple locations at increasing rates. Such plans should be based on a formal, well-conceived strategy to enhance customer access, reduce operational costs, and minimize ongoing capital investments by planning flexible, multiuse space. Although future expansion may be planned for emergency departments (EDs) or interventional imaging services, many hospital-based departments are being downsized because of the shift of treatments and procedures to the point of care. With increasingly miniaturized and mobile equipment (such as tabletop lab test analyzers and portable digital imaging units) and the gravitation of services to the physicians' office as equipment (such as ultrasound and electrocardiogram devices) becomes less costly to acquire, large, centralized departments need reconfiguration. With the high cost of the most advanced, floor-mounted imaging equipment—such as computed tomography, positron emission tomography, and magnetic resonance imaging scanners—departments are often expected to schedule patients on extended shifts and weekends, thus increasing workload capacity significantly without an increase in space.

Because of the many current issues associated with diagnostic and treatment services on the hospital campus, the senior leadership team should define specific strategies and actions to guide ongoing investments in facility upgrading and acquisition of new technology and medical equipment.

## Outpatient Services Configuration and Provision of Physician Office Space

Most healthcare organizations require a focused facility investment strategy that corresponds to their market strategies for penetrating target markets and increasing market share, fostering physician recruitment, developing centers of excellence, and so on. The facility development strategy may address construction of freestanding, community-based urgent care centers; new outpatient facilities in partnership with surgeons or physician specialists; expansion or construction of physician office space on the hospital campus; or expansion of existing space for new or growing programs or services.

In particular, hospital leadership may develop a strategy to move high-volume, routine outpatient services off-site to less costly and more easily accessible facilities. This approach also reduces traffic and congestion on the main hospital campus and frees parking spaces. Examples include outpatient physical therapy, dialysis, and primary care clinics.

## Building Infrastructure Upgrading and Equipment Acquisition or Replacement

Unless a specific healthcare facility has been replaced in the recent decade, a strategy is generally required to address the need for continued maintenance and updating of the physical plant as facilities are retooled and renewed to meet changing demand and technology. The acquisition or replacement of new equipment are also frequently part of a long-range facility investment strategy and should be integrated with the organization's IT strategic plan.

## Patient Experience Improvement

In an effort to promote customer loyalty, provide a healing environment, and satisfy employers and payers, most healthcare organizations include some aspect of improving the patient's experience as one of their facility investment strategies. This goal may involve improving wayfinding and access to necessary services, colocating related services to provide one-stop shopping, upgrading the interior decor, or offering enhanced amenities. I have found that an understanding of the following points is key to improving the patient's experience.

### All Patients Are Not the Same

Healthcare customers tend to simply be categorized as inpatients or outpatients. However, as inpatients vary from the acutely ill with life-threatening conditions to short-stay patients undergoing routine procedures, outpatients range from those seeking care for life-threatening conditions to those focusing on fitness and wellness. They therefore have different needs and expectations, as shown in exhibit 6.1. At the same time, the distinction between an inpatient and an outpatient is blurring with new care delivery models, alternate care settings, and technological advances. Today, unless admitted through the ED, most patients arrive at the hospital as outpatients and are generally admitted postprocedure. With the explosion of minimally invasive surgery and same-day medical procedures, the only difference between an inpatient and an outpatient is often the length of their recovery—for example, four,

**Exhibit 6.1 Different Types of Outpatients**

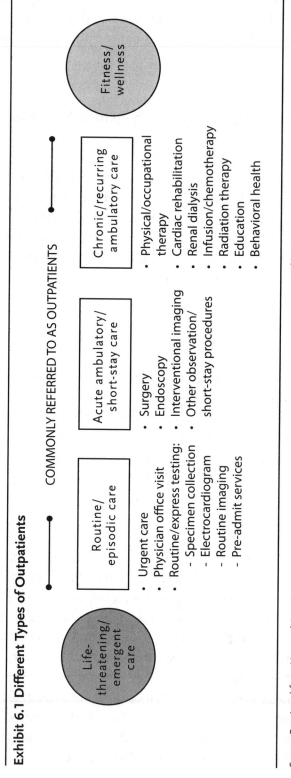

COMMONLY REFERRED TO AS OUTPATIENTS

Life-threatening/emergent care

**Routine/episodic care**
- Urgent care
- Physician office visit
- Routine/express testing:
  - Specimen collection
  - Electrocardiogram
  - Routine imaging
  - Pre-admit services

**Acute ambulatory/short-stay care**
- Surgery
- Endoscopy
- Interventional imaging
- Other observation/short-stay procedures

**Chronic/recurring ambulatory care**
- Physical/occupational therapy
- Cardiac rehabilitation
- Renal dialysis
- Infusion/chemotherapy
- Radiation therapy
- Education
- Behavioral health

Fitness/wellness

*Source:* Reprinted from Hayward (2015).

six, or eight hours versus a 30-hour stay or next-day discharge. These patients experience the same reception and intake processes and require the same predischarge instructions regardless of whether they are classified as an inpatient or outpatient.

Various types of care for outpatients include the following:

- Emergency or urgent care that requires immediate treatment for life-threatening conditions as well as care for patients who consider themselves to be in immediate need
- Routine or episodic care that may involve an occasional or once-a-year visit to the healthcare campus for routine care, such as an annual physical or a chest X-ray
- Acute ambulatory or short-stay care that may involve a once-in-a-lifetime experience, such as outpatient surgery or outpatient cardiac catheterization
- Chronic or recurring ambulatory care that involves frequent or ongoing visits—multiple times per week or month—for services such as physical therapy, cancer care, and dialysis
- Fitness and wellness activities that may include exercise regimens and health education for individuals who do not perceive themselves as patients

Each type of outpatient has different needs and expectations relative to site access and wayfinding, convenience, recognition by staff, education, and discharge instructions. Planners also need to consider the sharing of space by people with different needs. The sight of recovering patients exercising in a cardiac rehabilitation area may be inspirational and reassuring for a patient undergoing a heart catheterization or presurgery testing for open-heart surgery. However, it may not be advisable to mix patients undergoing chemotherapy with healthy patients undergoing annual health screening procedures.

### Separating Perception from Reality

Many factors affect the patient's and staff's perceptions of inadequate facilities, as shown in exhibit 6.2. Understanding the actual facility issues before investing millions of dollars in renovation or new construction is important. The initial first impression is also important, which is why the hospitality industry invests so many dollars in entrance facades and entry lobbies. A patient may also have different perceptions and expectations depending on his age, socioeconomic status, cultural background, education, and exposure to the media. However, the patient's perception of high-quality care may require more than contemporary, state-of-the-art facilities. Good design should also facilitate efficient processes, eliminate clutter, and create a productive work environment for care providers. Staff attitudes may ultimately affect patient satisfaction more than facilities.

### Improving the Patient Experience Does Not Always Mean Higher Costs

Acute care hospitals have been traditionally organized around departments rather than the patients' needs. In addition to the customer service center and express-testing concepts described in chapter 4, other new models for delivering services to the patient result in a win–win situation by achieving improved customer satisfaction and reduced costs. Examples include the following:

- Organizing patients by specialty rather than by acuity level and colocating a comprehensive range of services for a specific patient diagnosis or medical condition, such as a heart center or geriatric center
- Creating acuity adaptable or universal patient rooms (further described in chapter 15)
- Investing in Internet-based information and communication systems that allow patients and their families access to information at any time while reducing the labor costs associated with information desks and call centers

---

**Exhibit 6.2 Perception of Inadequate Facilities**

Operational/
information systems
problems?

Code/
regulatory
noncompliances?

Customer service/
marketing
issues?

Physical
plant/
HVAC
problems?

Inconvenient
location?

Perception of
inadequate
facilities

Image/
interior design
concerns?

Inappropriate
functional
layout?

Equipment/
technology
constraints?

Inadequate
signage?

Inappropriate
traffic mix?

---

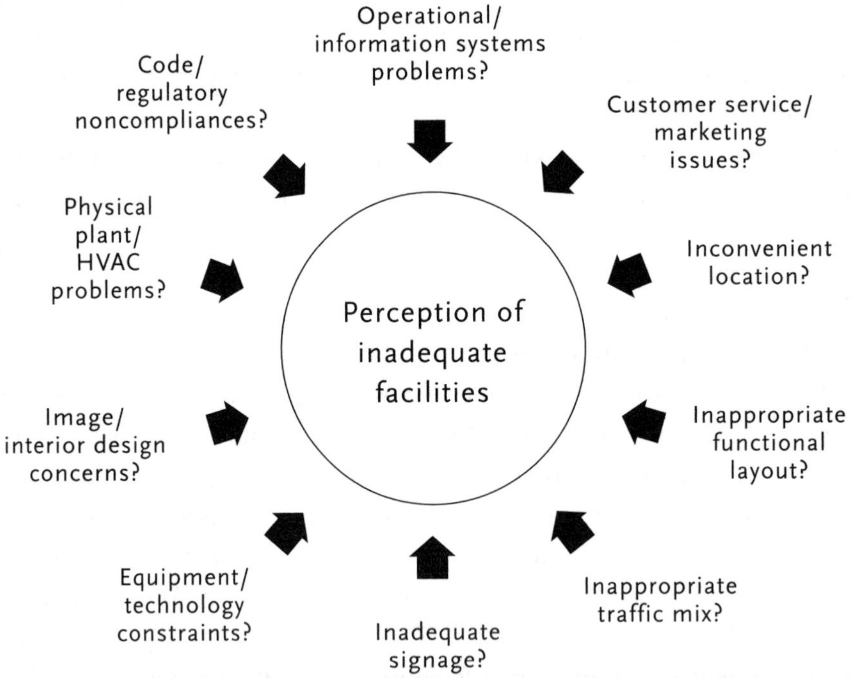

*Source*: Reprinted Hayward (2015).

### Improving the Patient Experience Begins Before Design

The goal of improving the patient's experience needs to be established and documented well before commencement of the design process. The integration of space programming and design into the organization's market strategy, clinical service line planning, operations redesign, and investments in new technology and information systems is critical to such improvement.

### The Patient Is Not the Only Customer

For an institution to be successful, it must consider other customers and their needs:

- *Family members and visitors* may have a more extensive exposure to the organization than the patient while they are parking, waiting during the procedure, and determining the patient's status at various points in time. The experience of family members and visitors may have a significant impact on the patient's perception.
- *Staff* may interact more positively with patients and their family members if they have a productive work environment and feel appreciated.
- *Employers* are demanding convenient access to services, a perception that the care is high quality, and cost-effective services for their employees.
- *Other major payers*, such as Medicare, demand cost-effective care.
- *Institutional partners* may require market branding, with a consistent quality of care and facility image at all service locations.

## Improving Wayfinding

Development of a simple and efficient wayfinding system to direct customers to their specific destination on the healthcare campus is a crucial part of any strategy for improving the patient's experience. Ease of navigation is becoming increasingly important in a competitive market with an aging and less ambulatory patient population. Wayfinding begins with the customer's arrival on the healthcare campus, and it involves signage and directional cues that assist the customer in parking, identifying the appropriate building entrance, and arriving at the desired service location. Key principles of wayfinding and signage for the healthcare campus include the following:

- A shopping center concept should be used, with an easily identifiable front door supported by dedicated entrances for customers who come frequently for a specific service.

- Customers should be able to see the front door before parking their cars—everyone wants to park adjacent to the front door, so not knowing where it is creates confusion and anxiety. In particular, I have found that directional signage in parking decks that orients the customer to the appropriate elevator and hospital entrance is frequently overlooked in the planning of signage systems.
- The customer service center concept should be implemented and located contiguous to the main entrance, using a hub-and-spoke model.
- A home base should be provided for families and visitors who may be arriving at different times to meet and gather, and appropriate amenities and communication systems should be available.
- Signage should serve the needs of patients and visitors; staff orientation should be done through in-service education.
- The number of potential destinations should be minimized; simple and logical names should be used for these destinations with a minimum amount of information to allow expedient decision making at any given intersection or decision node—for example, a diagnostic center as a single destination rather than separate signs for radiology, nuclear medicine, and ultrasound.
- Signage should be consistent with constant reinforcement; this repetition is particularly important when travel distances are lengthy. Intermittent seating should also be provided.
- Directional signage should be supplemented with architectural cues such as different floor coverings, ceiling heights, water features, statues, and dominant artwork that can be easily remembered and recalled to assist in orientation at any given point.

The development of a wayfinding program and a budget should occur in conjunction with immediate, short-term, and long-range facility reconfiguration strategies. A single administrative person should be responsible for signage and wayfinding, and a formal process should be in place for requesting new signs and for their approval, ensuring consistency with the facility master plan.

## Other Strategies

Depending on an organization's unique situation, the senior leadership team may develop additional strategies, such as the following:

- Relocate administrative offices outside the hospital to less costly and flexible space; an off-campus location may be chosen to free up parking and reduce traffic congestion on the hospital campus.
- Relocate or consolidate selected building support services into a modernized but less costly facility; an off-campus location may be considered that can support more than one hospital site—such as a warehouse, laundry, or kitchen—or a decision may be made to outsource specific services.
- Acquire land to enlarge the current campus to replace or renew aging buildings or wings, provide additional parking, or construct a new physician office building or specialty center.

Exhibit 6.3 provides an example of a healthcare organization's key investment strategies and the corresponding actions (tasks) required for implementation of one of the strategies.

## WHAT ABOUT PLANNING CENTERS OF EXCELLENCE?

Decisions to develop specific centers of excellence are complicated. An organization needs to initially understand the specific physical and virtual elements that

**Exhibit 6.3 Example: Community Hospital's Long-Range Facility Investment Strategies**

Strategy 1: Create a state-of-the-art emergency center.

Strategy 2: Unbundle nonclinical space from the hospital.

Strategy 3: Upgrade patient care units.

Strategy 4: Upgrade selected clinical services.

Strategy 5: Improve customer access to amenities.

Strategy 6: Upgrade building infrastructure and parking.

Strategy 7: Acquire additional property as available.

1.1 Expand/reconfigure the current ED to the west:
- Retain the current ambulance entry and access on the south adjacent to the trauma resuscitation area.
- Construct a new fast-track and emergent care area to the west with a new walk-in entry.
- Renovate a portion of the existing ED space for staff support and administrative offices.
- Redeploy the remaining (east) portion of the existing ED for expansion of other clinical services.

1.2 Provide a drive-up canopy for the new walk-in entry with adjacent, dedicated parking.

1.3 Maintain convenient access between the ED and the existing psychiatric observation unit.

give customers the perception of a "center" and to then identify which functional components and services will need to be physically adjacent versus virtually and electronically connected. Unless the new center is constructed as a freestanding facility on a new site, some physical components could be located in existing space, while others could be in a new addition. The trade-offs between paying for the initial capital and ongoing operational costs of achieving physical adjacency and settling for less-than-perfect convenience for the customer need to be reviewed and weighed carefully. The potential for increased revenue; reimbursement issues; and the demands of donors, partners, or investors may also affect the requirements of the physical design. Physicians often have difficulty imagining a center that is not an imposing edifice or at least a freestanding building. From the patients' perspective, once they arrive at a well-identified entrance and are greeted by a friendly and competent receptionist, they are generally oblivious to where they are treated as long as they are not asked to walk a great distance. Customers do not consider an elevator ride with a short walk to space in an existing building a hardship, even though the physician leaders may feel that new construction is mandatory.

## THE CHALLENGE OF PRIVATE DONORS

Every healthcare organization is delighted to have a private donor fund a building project. However, sometimes the donor has no interest in the organization's long-range capital investment strategy but wants to construct a building or fund a program that is not even on its radar screen. Most institutions are not in a position to reject such donations, and it is a rare administrator who has the backbone to turn down money rather than to compromise the organization's long-range facility development plan. Do not be deluded into thinking there are no strings attached to donor money. These projects can become difficult and emotionally draining. It helps, though, if the fundraising arm of the organization is integrated with the facility planning process in such a way that the organization can seek donations that are aligned with its long-range facility master plan. Most important, the real issue associated with constructing an unnecessary or oversized building is affording the ongoing operational costs, even though the initial construction is financed by someone else (Waite 2005).

## IS "DOING NOTHING" A STRATEGY?

Board members may commonly ask, what happens if we do nothing? Inaction may appear to be a viable strategy for an organization that is looking for a merger partner or trying to conserve capital to build a replacement facility. However, differentiating between doing nothing and maintaining the status quo is important. Just to maintain the status quo and ensure that market share does not erode and that key staff do not leave, money will need to be spent to maintain critical building systems and to upgrade furnishings and finishes to uphold a clean and professional image.

## FUTURE FACILITY CONFIGURATION DRAWINGS

Once the senior leadership team has reached consensus on future strategies and corresponding actions, the facility planner can prepare future department location drawings that show the size and location of all departments at the conclusion of the proposed renovation, reconfiguration, new construction, or demolition. They may be highlighted graphically to illustrate phasing stages over time as appropriate. A site plan may also be required that illustrates proposed changes to site access, circulation, building entry points, designated parking areas, and new additions or replacement facilities. Supplemental diagrams and graphics are frequently used as communication tools, such as the building section, or stacking, diagrams described in chapter 2. An example of a typical future department location drawing is illustrated in exhibit 6.4. Depending on the abilities of your in-house resources, such as your in-house architect, and whether you are using outside assistance from a predesign planning consultant, you may need to involve a design consultant at this point to perform a feasibility study, particularly if you anticipate major facility expansion. This study may include an analysis of alternative siting options, horizontal or vertical expansion trade-offs, and facility reuse issues. However, most predesign planning consultants, who specialize in facility master planning, will have licensed architects on their staff to routinely assist with the translation of your facility development strategies into facility reconfiguration actions (or options as applicable) in conjunction with strategy development.

## REFERENCE

Hayward, C. 2015. *SpaceMed Guide: A Space Planning Guide for Healthcare Facilities*, 3rd ed. Ann Arbor, MI: HA Ventures.

Waite, P. S. 2005. *The Non-Architect's Guide to Major Capital Projects: Planning, Designing, and Delivering New Buildings*. Ann Arbor, MI: Society for College and University Planning.

# Exhibit 6.4 Example: Future Department Location Drawing

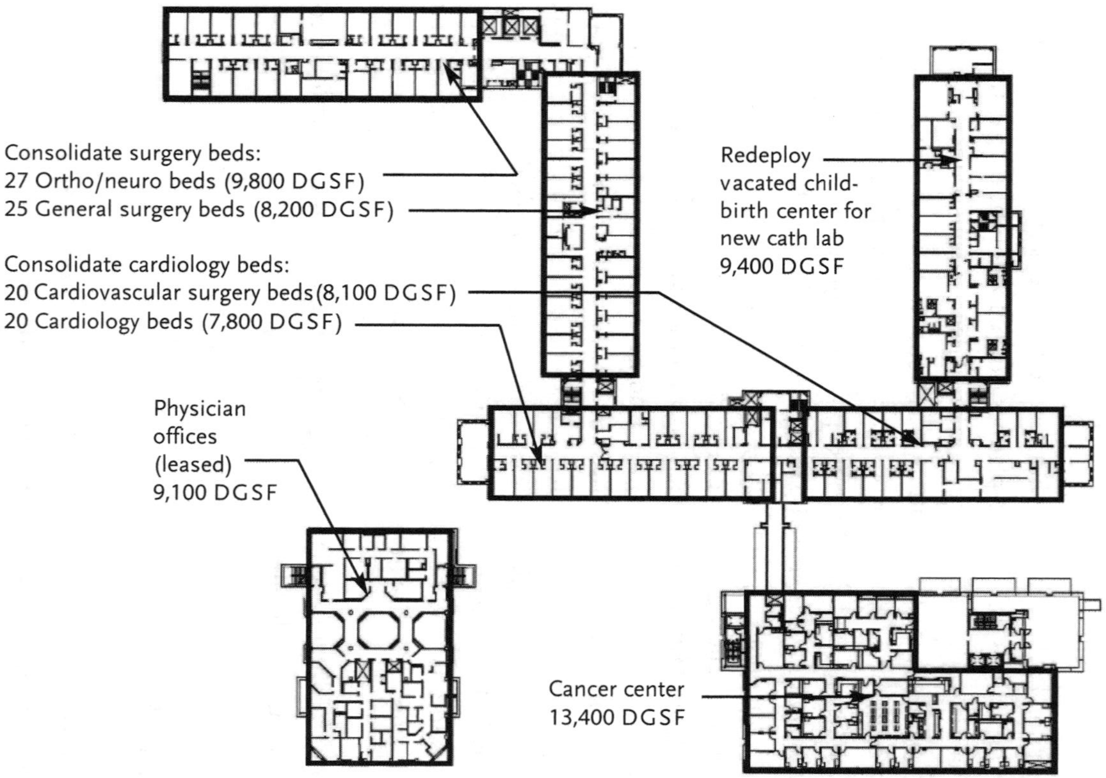

Redeploy vacated child-birth center for new cath lab 9,400 DGSF

Cancer center 13,400 DGSF

Consolidate surgery beds:
27 Ortho/neuro beds (9,800 DGSF)
25 General surgery beds (8,200 DGSF)

Consolidate cardiology beds:
20 Cardiovascular surgery beds (8,100 DGSF)
20 Cardiology beds (7,800 DGSF)

Physician offices (leased) 9,100 DGSF

# CHAPTER 7

# Identifying Specific Projects and Preparing a Phasing and Implementation Plan

ONCE CONSENSUS HAS been reached on a long-range facility investment plan, hospital leadership can commence the translation of the strategies and corresponding actions into defined projects. The rationale for specific renovation, expansion, or new construction projects undertaken by healthcare organizations may not always appear logical or prudent, given limited capital dollars. Most hospital leaders, care providers, facility planners, and architects can cite an example of a misguided project—almost always by some other organization or under the direction of someone else. Today, most healthcare organizations have many more demands for facility upgrading and expansion than available dollars—particularly when bricks-and-mortar projects compete with investments in new medical equipment and information technology and with lenders providing their own scrutiny.

## DEVELOPING A RATIONAL APPROACH

Healthcare leaders may consider a number of factors to reach consensus about which projects ultimately get funded and the sequence of their funding compared to other capital expenditures. At a minimum, they should evaluate the rationale for each potential project on the basis of the following factors:

- *Mitigate risk and improve health safety.* Facility issues related to building code deficiencies, patient safety, or compliance with other regulatory requirements are usually the highest priorities as funding decisions are being made.
- *Increase revenue.* Expanding the capacity of existing services—where there is clear evidence of pent-up demand—is almost always a high priority.

- *Enhance operational efficiency.* The ability of a specific project to deliver an immediate return on investment, such as a reduction in labor costs or a minimization of investments in new medical equipment and instrumentation, will be viewed positively by potential lenders.
- *Improve space use.* A one-time capital investment to consolidate space or improve the use of existing space (thus increasing capacity) will reduce the associated costs for housekeeping, maintenance, utilities, and other ongoing facility-related costs.
- *Improve customer access and satisfaction.* Depending on the market dynamics, competition from other community providers, and the organization's mission, improving patient access and customer satisfaction can result in additional market share (and revenue).
- *Build future capacity.* This rationale may be appropriate for a project in a growing market or where another competitor could potentially go out of business—resulting in an opportunity to increase market share.
- *Renew or retool the physical plant.* Every business—whether in healthcare or any other industry—must routinely invest in its physical plant to stay competitive as its business model evolves. For healthcare, these changes are occurring in medical practice, reimbursement, regulations, technology, and customer preferences.
- *Facilitate donor and partner funding.* A project may quickly become a high priority when a donor is ready and willing to fund all or part of a specific project. At the same time, a partner may be identified who can share in the funding (and, more important, in the ongoing operational costs).

The matrix in exhibit 7.1 provides an example used by a senior leadership team to summarize its target projects and the corresponding rationale for each. Cells with an *X* indicate the potential rationale for a specific project on the list. Readers should note that each healthcare organization will have a unique rationale for any given project.

Once the senior leadership team has reached consensus on the rationale for each project, specific projects can be grouped and sequenced on the following bases:

- Urgency (e.g., in response to a competitive threat, code issues, or revenue generation)
- Renovation or construction feasibility and cost-effectiveness (i.e., the sequencing of tasks)
- Availability of capital at different points in time
- Ability of the organization to handle multiple ongoing projects

**Exhibit 7.1 Example: Summarizing Target Projects and Rationale in a Matrix**

| | Mitigate Risk/Improve Health Safety | Increase Revenue | Enhance Operational Efficiency | Improve Space Use | Improve Customer Access/Satisfaction | Build Future Capacity | Renew/Retool the Physical Plant | Facilitate Donor/Partner Funding |
|---|---|---|---|---|---|---|---|---|
| Expand the emergency department | | | | X | | | | |
| Renovate the main surgery suite | | X | | | | | | |
| Expand the pharmacy | | X | | | X | X | | X |
| Replace the kitchen | | X | | | | X | | X |
| Create a time-share clinic | X | X | | | | | X | X |
| Reconfigure the laboratory | X | X | | | X | | | X |
| Demolish the old nursing school | | X | X | | X | X | | X |

The detailed phasing and implementation plan lists each project, the required sequencing, and the corresponding capital needs over time. Many types of project planning and management software are available to track each specific project's actual expected start date, completion date, and person responsible for its oversight. Exhibit 7.2 provides an example of a summary format used by a senior leadership team to communicate projects and dollars as part of the funding approval process.

## GROUPING OF PROJECTS BY PRIORITY

Projects are generally grouped according to their priority as follows:

- *Immediate priority* is for projects that must be completed as soon as possible (even though renovation or construction may take up to two years).
- *Short-term priority* is for projects that must be completed in two to five years and for which planning needs to be initiated promptly
- *Long-range priority* is for projects where completion will be needed beyond five years, after the immediate and short-term projects have been completed. The need for these projects would generally be reconfirmed at some point during the initial five-year time frame and may be based on achievement of critical benchmarks.
- *Independent* projects may also be identified. Such projects might qualify if their timing and completion is relatively independent from other projects. In

# Exhibit 7.2 Example: Detailed Project Phasing and Implementation Plan

| Task | Project | Pre-task | Site | 2016 | 2017 | 2018 | 2019 | 2020 | 2021 | 2022 | 2023 | 2024 | 2025 | Total |
|------|---------|----------|------|------|------|------|------|------|------|------|------|------|------|-------|
| 1.1 | Relocate plant operations (3M) | — | MSH | $0.50 | | | | | | | | | | $0.50 |
| 1.2 | Consolidate home health (leased) | — | Off | tbd | | | | | | | | | | $0.00 |
| 1.3 | Demolish White Building | 1.1 | MSH | $0.50 | | | | | | | | | | $0.50 |
| 1.4 | Create new parking spaces | 1.3 | MSH | $0.40 | | | | | | | | | | $0.40 |
| 2.1 | Convert 5N to office occupancy | — | MSH | | $2.00 | | | | | | | | | $2.00 |
| 2.2 | Relocate IS (NE to 5N) | 2.1 | MSH | $0.20 | | | | | | | | | | $0.20 |
| 2.3 | Relocate volunteers (NE to CB) | 4.5 | MSH | $0.20 | | | | | | | | | | $0.20 |
| 2.4 | Demolish NE wing | 2.3 | MSH | | $0.35 | | | | | | | | | $0.35 |
| 2.5 | Create new parking spaces | 2.4 | MSH | | $0.40 | | | | | | | | | $0.40 |
| 3.1 | Create customer service center | 4.2 | MSH | | $2.40 | | | | | | | | | $2.40 |
| 3.2 | Upgrade surgery suite (2E) | 3.1 | MSH | | | $4.50 | | | | | | | | $4.50 |
| 3.3 | Create ICU/CCU beds (2W) | 3.2 | MSH | | | | $2.00 | | | | | | | $2.00 |
| 3.4 | Convert 7/8N to office occupancy | 3.3 | MSH | | | | | $3.10 | | | | | | $3.10 |
| 3.5 | Reconfigure OP services (1st floor) | 3.1 | MSH | | | $4.00 | | | | | | | | $4.00 |
| 3.6 | Convert 4M for neuro unit | 3.4 | MSH | | | | | | $5.00 | | | | | $5.00 |
| 3.7 | Upgrade 2M (ortho) | 3.6 | MSH | | | | | | | $2.00 | | | | $2.00 |
| 3.8 | Convert 3M for oncology unit | 3.6 | MSH | | | | | | | $6.30 | | | | $6.30 |
| 3.9 | Convert 6N to office occupancy | 3.8 | MSH | | | | | | | | $1.20 | $1.20 | | $2.40 |
| 3.10 | Demolish CB/improve facade | 3.9 | MSH | | | | | | $2.20 | | | | | $2.20 |

Preliminary Estimated Project Cost (in Millions)

# Exhibit 7.2 Example: Detailed Project Phasing and Implementation Plan (*Continued*)

Preliminary Estimated Project Cost (in Millions)

| Task | Project | Pre-task | Site | 2016 | 2017 | 2018 | 2019 | 2020 | 2021 | 2022 | 2023 | 2024 | 2025 | Total |
|---|---|---|---|---|---|---|---|---|---|---|---|---|---|---|
| 4.1 | Upgrade surgery/recovery | — | CCH | $2.50 | | | | | | | | | | $2.50 |
| 4.2 | Convert 2N to generic/business office | 4.1 | CCH | $2.70 | | | | | | | | | | $2.70 |
| 4.3 | Upgrade ED | — | CCH | $3.20 | | | | | | | | | | $3.20 |
| 4.4 | Upgrade selected clinical services | — | CCH | $2.70 | $2.70 | | | | | | | | | $5.40 |
| 4.5 | Consolidate HR (1M) | 1.2 | CCH | | $0.50 | | | | | | | | | $0.50 |
| 4.6 | Consolidate laboratory | 4.5 | CCH | | $1.20 | | | | | | | | | $1.20 |
| 4.7 | Upgrade 2E/W | — | CCH | | | $1.50 | | | | | | | | $1.50 |
| | Total project cost | | | $12.90 | $9.55 | $10.00 | $2.00 | $3.10 | $7.20 | $8.30 | $1.20 | $1.20 | $0.00 | $55.45 |

some cases, the senior leadership team may establish specific benchmarks that would trigger implementation (such as a census increase over multiple fiscal quarters, certificate-of-need submittal by a competitor, or donor funding).

## DEVELOPING PRELIMINARY PROJECT COST ESTIMATES

During the predesign planning stage, limited information is available regarding construction conditions, the anticipated quality of construction, the construction bidding climate, and other factors that could influence the total project cost. Although establishing an early order-of-magnitude estimate for the cost of construction or renovation is necessary, estimates made at this time should be regarded with caution. Typically, the process for developing a preliminary cost estimate includes first estimating the *base construction cost* and then applying a series of factors or additional budget items to estimate the *total project cost.*

To estimate the base cost of renovation, the anticipated cost of new construction can be factored:

- *Minor renovation* includes construction with minimal demolition of existing walls and use of existing utilities and is usually 25–35 percent of the cost of new construction.
- *Moderate renovation* assumes the reuse of the primary mechanical systems, with some demolition of existing walls, and is usually 50–60 percent of the cost of new construction.
- *Major renovation* assumes the complete demolition of the existing walls and major reworking of the mechanical systems and is generally around 75 percent of the cost of new construction. However, some major renovation may actually be equal to or greater than the cost of new construction.

Base construction cost estimates are calculated and totaled for all facility components included in the project using either department gross square feet (if the project includes the renovation of specific departments) or building gross square feet (if the project includes new construction).

Once the base construction cost is estimated, the total project cost can be estimated by budgeting additional dollars for the following:

- Site work can be estimated at 10 percent for new construction.
- Multilevel parking can be estimated at around $18,000 per car (Cudney 2015) while underground parking may be 40–60 percent higher—not

including the cost of land acquisition, project-related fees, and other soft costs.

- Moveable equipment, furniture, and furnishings are some of the most difficult elements to estimate during predesign planning and may vary from 10 percent to 40 percent of the base construction cost, depending on factors such as the extent of equipment to be reused and vendor discounts. Typically, major imaging equipment is purchased separately from the construction budget and is therefore accounted for separately. Alternately, a single dollar figure can be budgeted or a list developed of specific major medical equipment items.
- A building and construction contingency factor of 10 percent is usually added to allow for unknown costs that cannot be identified at the start of construction.
- Project-related fees for programming consultants, architects, equipment planners, construction managers, interior designers, and so on may total 10–15 percent of the base construction cost.
- Other costs—such as land acquisition, testing and inspections, administrative and legal fees, and financing costs—should be added as appropriate.

An *inflation factor* may need to be added to adjust the base construction cost to reflect future construction conditions. Most contractors will adjust their construction estimates to the midpoint of construction to account for anticipated inflation in labor and materials if the project is large and will be constructed over a multiyear period.

## DIFFERENTIATING BETWEEN BASE CONSTRUCTION COSTS AND PROJECT COSTS

After additional costs for these factors are tabulated, they should be added to the base construction cost to arrive at the total project cost. Just as confusing net and gross space can lead to misunderstandings (as described in chapter 2), confusing the base construction cost and project cost can also lead to problems. Facility planners, architects, and even construction specialists often refer to "cost" without qualifying whether it is simply the base construction cost or the total amount that must be funded (project cost). This vagueness can be disastrous because the project cost may be 50–70 percent higher than the base construction cost.

# PREPARING REALISTIC COST ESTIMATES: A CATCH-22

The preparation of a project cost estimate at the predesign (and schematic design) stage often presents a catch-22 in which the desired outcome is difficult to attain because of inherent but well-intentioned conflicts of interest. Project cost estimates may be provided by one or more people involved in the facility planning process, including the architect, the construction manager, a professional cost estimator, the hospital-based facility manager, or a facility planning or project management consultant.

If asked to prepare the project cost estimate, an architect who may eventually be awarded the design contract may understate the complexity and cost of the project for fear that the project might be derailed or downsized and the design concept jeopardized. A construction manager who may eventually be charged with delivering the completed project on budget may provide an overly conservative estimate. Construction managers are most comfortable and confident with providing cost estimates based on a set of detailed architectural drawings and specifications, and they naturally overcompensate when only limited information concerning a potential project is available. If the project cost estimate is too high, the potential project may be deemed infeasible or literally sent "back to the drawing board." Valuable staff time and professional fees are wasted when the project is appropriate and affordable but derailed because of a conservatively high cost estimate. The same thing can happen when the project cost is understated and requires redesign midstream, resulting in expensive *change orders*.

This push–pull situation can be modulated with an adept facility manager who has experience at the particular healthcare facility. A hospital-based facility manager can provide historical comparisons based on previous renovation or construction projects at the specific campus. A knowledge of unique construction conditions, the quality of construction anticipated by the organization's leadership, and the organization's corporate culture regarding decision making have a major impact on the accuracy of early predesign project cost estimates. At the predesign planning stage, professional cost estimators will have little to contribute and, like construction specialists, may be overly conservative. Input from an experienced facility planning consultant will provide objectivity and will help an organization focus on the broader question: Can the specific organization implement its immediate and short-term projects with the available capital resources? As the facility planning process progresses and the level of detail increases, some projects will require more money, but others will require less, so that the overall budget will be appropriate.

Ultimately, a healthcare organization should hire planning, design, and construction professionals who can assist the owner in getting the best project within a fixed budget by evaluating trade-offs and weighing advantages and disadvantages.

Such deliberations may range from decisions related to operational concepts and their impact on staffing, equipment, and space needs to evaluating alternative architectural design solutions and comparing trade-offs between the quality and the quantity of space.

## PLANNING A NEW FACILITY FROM THE GROUND UP

The planning of a replacement hospital or a new freestanding healthcare facility requires a different approach because the entire facility becomes the project. Although in some cases phased construction may be planned, a master project budget is generally developed that addresses all aspects of the project from start to completion. John Kemper's 2010 book *Launching a Capital Facility Project* provides an example of a sample master project budget that addresses the costs associated with the planning, design, and construction of a new or replacement healthcare facility.

## REFERENCES

Cudney, G. 2015. "Parking Structure Cost Outlook for 2015." *Carl Walker.* Accessed September 14. www.carlwalker.com/wp-content/uploads/2015/07/Carl-Walker-2015-Cost-Article.pdf.

Kemper, J. E. 2010. *Launching a Capital Facility Project: A Guide for Healthcare Leaders,* 2nd ed. Chicago: Health Administration Press.

# CHAPTER 8

# Beginning Detailed Operational and Space Programming

DETAILED OPERATIONAL (FUNCTIONAL) and space programming begins once a specific project has been defined, approved, and funded. This final stage of the predesign planning process generally begins once consensus has been reached on an appropriate long-range facility investment strategy and a phasing and implementation plan has been prepared. Detailed operational and space programs should be prepared for immediate or short-term projects for which planning needs to commence. This process provides a forum for rethinking operational processes and the use of technology in such a way that facility investments enhance operational efficiency and improve customer service, in addition to providing newer, code-compliant, and aesthetically pleasing facilities. After administrative approval, the operational and space program becomes an "approved" document serving as a control mechanism for all members of the planning and design team during the schematic drawing and design development phases of the architectural design process. The operational and space programming document should provide all necessary information for the design architect to begin schematic design.

## DEFINING OPERATIONAL AND SPACE PROGRAMMING

Operational and space programming, as defined today, includes the two-step process of documenting the operational (functional) planning assumptions and preparing a detailed space listing (space program). Traditionally, a list of spaces and their corresponding sizes was the only written documentation preceding facility design. Today, operational planning precedes space planning, and one document—the operational and space program—combines the results of both processes. Although the terms *functional and space programming* and *functional space programming* are commonly used, I prefer to use the term *operational and space programming* throughout this book to emphasize the rigor that should be involved at this critical point in the facility planning process.

The tasks necessary to developing a detailed operational and space program are among the most critical in the facility development process. From my experience, long-term operational costs often exceed the initial capital cost of renovation and construction in a couple of years. Efficient planning at this stage will save significant operational dollars in the future. Also, paying careful attention to the development of realistic workload projections and differentiating between actual space needs and wish lists will guard against the construction of inappropriate and inflexible space and will eliminate overbuilding.

## COMPONENTS OF THE OPERATIONAL PROGRAM

The operational program should provide a description of the scope of services and operational concepts as well as the numbers and categories of people, systems, and equipment necessary to operate the specific department or service line at a projected workload level. The operational program should also address facility layout considerations, necessary and desired physical proximities, and opportunities to achieve operational flexibility and accommodate future growth. Although the outline can be tailored to meet an organization's specific situation, typical components of the operational program are described in the following sections, along with sample text that illustrates the scope and level of detail that should be provided.

## EXAMPLE: OPERATIONAL PROGRAM FOR AN ENDOSCOPY SUITE

### Current Situation (Baseline)

The current scope of services, space allocation, and location should be identified, and deficiencies requiring correction should be documented.

> Mercy Medical Center currently operates two endoscopy suites. One is located on the second floor of the Ambulatory Care Center (ACC) on the Mercy Medical main campus, and the other is located on the third floor of the Mercy East Campus hospital.

- *ACC.* This suite currently has seven procedure rooms and occupies approximately 4,580 department gross square feet (DGSF). The staff only use six rooms because one of the procedure rooms is small and difficult to use. The suite also has 12 patient prep and recovery bays that are undersized, with limited space for patient nourishment, linens, supply storage, and trash holding. Endoscopic retrograde cholangiopancreatography (ERCP) is done in a dedicated fluoroscopy room in the main radiology department. Bronchoscopies are performed in the pulmonary lab with nursing coverage provided by the endoscopy department.
- *Mercy East.* This endoscopy suite is composed of five procedure rooms (four endoscopy and one bronchoscopy) occupying 4,470 DGSF. The rooms are adequately sized, with contiguous patient toilet rooms. Patient prep and recovery functions occur in the shared 30-bed ambulatory recovery area on the fourth floor of the hospital.

## Future Vision and Planning Goals

Strategic (market) planning and operational performance improvement goals pertaining to the specific department or service line should be specified to keep the planning team focused on the expected results.

Mercy Medical is considering consolidation of the endoscopy suite located on the third floor of Mercy East hospital with the endoscopy suite located on the second floor of the ACC on the Mercy Medical main campus. The consolidated suite will likely continue to be located on the second floor of the ACC. Adjacent expansion space is potentially available because of the recently vacated dialysis unit (5,350 DGSF); other adjacent space currently used for private physician offices could also be relocated.

Other assumptions include the following:

- Outpatient registration will continue to occur on the first floor of the ACC, and patients will then proceed to the second floor endoscopy waiting area.
- Bronchoscopy procedures will be consolidated at Mercy Medical as well. These procedures will continue to be done in the pulmonary lab with nursing coverage provided by the endoscopy staff.
- ERCPs will eventually be moved to the consolidated endoscopy suite with the timing dependent on replacement of the existing unit. In the short term, ERCPs will continue to occur in the main radiology department on the first floor of Mercy Medical.

## Current and Projected Workloads

A detailed analysis of the current and future workloads for patient care functions can involve evaluation of case mix and scheduling patterns as well as the interrelationship between the volume and timing of arrivals, desirable waiting times, and the number of procedure rooms or workstations. Identification of average and peak workloads is particularly important for those services whose workload is primarily a random occurrence, such as emergency visits and obstetrics deliveries.

At Mercy Medical, a total of 12,096 patients received gastroscopy or bronchoscopy procedures in 2014:

- 9,222 procedures at the Mercy Medical ACC (8,853 gastroscopies and 369 bronchoscopies)
- 2,874 procedures at Mercy East (2,759 gastroscopies and 115 bronchoscopies)

Approximately 55 percent of the total procedures are colonoscopies and 30 percent are gastrointestinal procedures. In addition, flexible sigmoidoscopies, ERCPs, esophageal motility testing, transesophageal echocardiography, 24-hour pH monitoring, and bronchoscopies are performed. Outpatient procedures represent 90 percent of the total volume. The combined workload is projected to grow at a rate of 1 percent per year, assuming that all physicians from Mercy East move toward consolidation at the Mercy Medical ACC.

Assuming an increase to approximately 12,200 procedures (excluding bronchoscopies) over the next five years, a total of six to seven procedure rooms and 14 prep and recovery cubicles are required. Seven procedure rooms have been programmed to provide the flexibility to include other procedures (e.g., bronchoscopies) in the future.

## Planned Hours of Operation

Assumptions regarding the planned hours of operation by daily shift and by days of the week should be specified.

Mercy Medical anticipates that the consolidated endoscopy service will operate approximately 12 hours per day, Monday through Friday, 5:30 am to 5:30 pm Procedures will generally be scheduled between 6:00 am and 3:00 pm, as well as on Saturdays (e.g., 8:00 am to 12:00 pm) if staff are available.

## Current and Future Staffing

The numbers, categories, and work scheduling patterns of people who will be working in the department should be documented. Staffing primarily affects the provision of administrative spaces such as offices, workstations, conference rooms, and lounges. Scheduling patterns are of particular importance in determining the number of people on the day (or primary) shift for which space is planned. Most important, the future types and numbers of full-time equivalents (FTEs) should be reviewed relative to projected future workloads to ensure that the new or expanded facilities do not require additional staffing that cannot be justified on the basis of workload growth.

A single manager currently oversees the combined department with team leaders at both sites. There are currently 28.95 FTEs (July payroll)—5.25 at Mercy East and 23.70 at the Mercy Medical ACC.

The proposed staffing for the consolidated department is estimated at 26.30 FTEs, resulting in a reduction of 2.65 FTEs even though the workload is expected to increase within five years (see following table).

### Staffing at Mercy Medical Center's Endoscopy Suites

| Position | Mercy East FTEs | ACC FTEs | Consolidated Staffing (Day Shift) |
|---|---|---|---|
| Manager | — | 1.0 | 1.0 |
| Team leader | 1.0 | 1.0 | 1.0 |
| Registered nurse | — | 1.0 | 1.0 |
| Specialty registered nurse I | 0.5 | 3.0 | 3.0 |
| Specialty registered nurse II | 1.0 | 1.9 | 2.5 |
| Specialty registered nurse III | — | 4.8 | 4.8 |
| Gastrointestinal (GI) technician | 2.75 | 5.0 | 7.0 |
| Lead GI tech specialist | — | 3.0 | 3.0 |
| Tech assistant I | — | 1.0 | 1.0 |
| Clerk receptionist | — | 1.0 | 1.0 |
| Surgical services assistant | — | 1.0 | 1.0 |
| **Total** | **5.25** | **23.7** | **26.3** |

## Equipment, Technology, and Support Systems

Major equipment items and support systems should be documented because of their impact on space need and capital requirements. Equipment units that take up floor space and other items that either represent a significant capital expense or have a direct effect on productivity should be identified. The significance of equipment and support systems will vary depending on the department or service line.

Equipment at the Mercy East and ACC endoscopy suites varies in age and usefulness:

- *Mercy East.* The scopes used in the four rooms at Mercy East are eight years old. The department is currently evaluating a lease option for Pentax scopes on the basis of a fee-per-procedure model. The existing equipment can be used as backup equipment.
- *ACC.* The Olympus scopes used in the six rooms at the Mercy Medical ACC are in good condition.

In summary, no additional endoscopy equipment will be required to accommodate the combined workload. The radiographic and fluoroscopic equipment in the procedure room used for ERCPs in the radiology department needs to be replaced. When the hospital acquires the newer model, the equipment will be installed in the consolidated endoscopy suite.

Assumptions regarding institution-wide support systems such as information technology (IT), central scheduling, and materials management should be documented and coordinated through central sources in the organization.

Preliminary operational assumptions for the consolidated endoscopy suite include the following:

- *Registration.* Patients are generally preregistered. Patients will complete registration and have insurance verified at the registration area on the first floor of the ACC.
- *Scheduling.* A centralized scheduling system is in place to optimize patient convenience and staff and physician workflow.
- *Cashiering.* Payments by credit card and check will be accepted at the point of service. Cash payments will be directed to the cashier in the Customer Service Center.
- *Telecommunications.* The central hospital switchboard will be used and supported by the Mercy Medical telecommunication system.
- *Information systems.* Order entry and results reporting will be fully automated using the existing system. Patient demographics and archives will

be available to support patient registration. Digital dictation will continue in the consolidated department using the outsourced Medquest system.

- *Health records.* Conversion to an electronic health record system has been completed. Any remaining patient charts will be stored at the nurse station and documentation area.
- *Linen.* Linen for the endoscopy suite will continue to be provided by the same contract linen service used by Mercy Medical and delivered to the department on routine and requisition bases. With the consolidation, the suite will need additional inventory.
- *Medications.* The endoscopy suite will be supported from the Mercy Medical pharmacy. Limited stock medications (narcotics, antibiotics, and so on) are kept in the suite. Ideally, a Pyxis unit should be used to track medications. (Mercy East currently uses Pyxis.)
- *Scope processing.* The endoscopy suite will continue to reprocess endoscopes. No central reprocessing of instruments at Mercy Medical, in support of the consolidated suite, is anticipated.
- *Supply storage.* The Mercy Medical materials management department will receive and store bulk supplies, which are delivered to the endoscopy suite in retail form on routine and requisition bases; supplies will be stocked on mobile carts.
- *Hazardous waste.* Hazardous waste will be bagged and held in the soiled utility areas until picked up by environmental services.
- *Patient transportation.* The endoscopy suite uses aides for transport of inpatients to and from nursing units.
- *Food.* The Mercy Medical kitchen will provide food service as needed (e.g., snacks for outpatients). Staff will use the food court on the second floor of the hospital, and a staff lounge or break room is provided in the department.
- *Parking.* Mercy Medical assumes that sufficient parking capacity will be available at the parking garage on the main campus to accommodate patients and visitors. Staff will continue to park in the staff parking lot, and physicians will continue to park in the physicians' parking lot.

## Functional Adjacencies and Access

For departments involved in direct patient care, patient access should be defined, including assumptions regarding site access, parking, building access points, and unique signage and wayfinding requirements. Optimal interdepartmental and intradepartmental functional adjacencies should also be noted.

Mercy Medical can continue to use the existing ACC reception and waiting area on the second floor, with nearby elevator access, although ideally it should be reconfigured or enlarged to accommodate the additional patient volume.

Outpatients will complete registration and check-in at the registration area on the first floor and then proceed to the second floor reception area of the consolidated suite. Outpatients will change in their prep cubicles and their belongings will be stored in lockers in central patient alcoves.

A corridor connection must be maintained on the second floor to facilitate circulation between the ACC elevators and the rest of the hospital complex (via the East Pavilion).

## Future Trends and Operational Flexibility

Planning uncertainties as a result of future trends should be identified, and opportunities to achieve flexibility should be noted as well.

Endoscopy workload fluctuations, physician scheduling patterns, and reimbursement changes should be closely monitored to detect their potential impact on future use of the Mercy Medical endoscopy suite. Because outpatients represent 90 percent of the current workload, the workload could fluctuate substantially over time depending on the physicians' continued interest in performing these procedures at Mercy Medical versus in their office suites.

## Outstanding Issues to Be Resolved

Issues that require additional input from senior management or physician leaders should be documented along with a time frame for resolution.

Bronchoscopies will continue to be performed in the pulmonary lab at Mercy Medical. Additional procedure room capacity may be needed in the endoscopy suite if it is decided that these procedures will be performed there. Bronchoscopy volume is projected to be approximately 500 per year (two patients per day).

Although adequate procedure space appears to be available for consolidating the services at the Mercy Medical campus, the existing suite is extremely deficient in support space. Relocating the prep and recovery functions to the vacated dialysis area (or other vacated space) and providing additional support space in the existing suite should be considered.

Although eventual relocation of the radiographic and fluoroscopic unit from the main radiology department to the endoscopy suite is planned, Mercy Medical should replace the equipment within two years. An additional procedure room has been programmed that can be shelled until the equipment is replaced and the decision to relocate this service to the endoscopy suite is confirmed.

Preparation of the operational program is typically an iterative process beginning with the accumulation of baseline data for the specific department or functional area to be programmed—for example, current and projected workloads, staffing, equipment, space allocation, and existing deficiencies. A listing of preliminary functional and operational assumptions can be developed for initial review by a designated task force charged with its development. The task force, or *user group*, should include department or service line leadership as well as other key stakeholders. The task force generally refines and finalizes the draft operational (functional) program narrative at subsequent meetings (typically three). At this point, the preparation of the space program can begin.

## PREPARING THE SPACE PROGRAM

Space programming is the process by which the operational program is translated into room-specific space requirements, and it can begin once the functional and operational planning assumptions are documented. The space program should provide a tabulation of every room or area required with the assigned function, number (or units), area needed for each unit to perform the function, and total area required for the function. Comments for each space should also be provided regarding the location of the space relative to other spaces, the minimum dimensions, the major equipment items to be accommodated in the space, and any special performance or environmental requirements as shown in exhibit 8.1.

Generally, the process begins with a list of spaces to be included for a selected department or functional area, proceeds to the preparation of a draft space program to be reviewed by the designated task force, and concludes with the approval of the space program by the task force members. Architectural design (schematic design) should only begin after task force members approve and sign off on the operational and space program.

**Exhibit 8.1 Example: Detailed Space Program**

| Room/Area | Units | NSF | Total NSF | Comments |
|---|---|---|---|---|
| Patient and reception area | 1 | 80 | 80 | Proximate to waiting room and entrance to procedure area |
| Patient and visitor lounge | 1 | 270 | 270 | Seating for up to 18 visitors, television, coffee station, coat rack |
| Interview and consult room | 1 | 100 | 100 | Includes seating for 6–8 people |
| Public toilet | 1 | 55 | 55 | Wheelchair accessible |
| **Subtotal (patient intake area)** | | | **505** | |
| Patient locker alcove | 1 | 60 | 60 | Purse or tote bag lockers |
| Exam and consult room | 1 | 120 | 120 | |
| Patient prep and recovery bay | 14 | 80 | 1,120 | |
| Patient toilet room | 3 | 55 | 165 | Wheelchair accessible |
| Endoscopy procedure room | 6 | 200 | 1,200 | |
| Procedure room (shelled) | 1 | 200 | 200 | Shelled for future use |
| Nurse station/documentation area | 1 | 180 | 180 | Charting station with view of recovery bays |
| Automated medication dispensing unit | 1 | 40 | 40 | Pyxis unit with access to sink, refrigerator, and double-locked storage |
| Nourishment alcove | 1 | 40 | 40 | Sink, refrigerator, and ice machine |
| Emergency equipment alcove | 1 | 15 | 15 | Located in recovery suite |
| Clean workroom | 1 | 100 | 100 | |
| Soiled workroom | 1 | 80 | 80 | Soiled linen and trash holding, floor sink |

**Exhibit 8.1 Example: Detailed Space Program** (*Continued*)

| Room/Area | Units | NSF | Total NSF | Comments |
|---|---|---|---|---|
| Clean linen cart alcove | 1 | 20 | 20 | Space for two linen carts |
| Equipment storage room | 1 | 175 | 175 | |
| Wheelchair and stretcher alcove | 2 | 30 | 60 | |
| Tech work area | 1 | 80 | 80 | |
| Physician viewing and reading room | 1 | 80 | 80 | |
| Scope cleaning and storage room | 1 | 240 | 240 | Includes decontamination area, clean work area, scope storage cabinet |
| Environmental services room | 1 | 40 | 40 | Space for service sink and cart |
| **Subtotal (procedure suite)** | | | **4,015** | |
| Private office (manager) | 1 | 100 | 100 | |
| Office (team leader) | 1 | 80 | 80 | |
| Staff lounge/break room | 1 | 180 | 180 | Provide counter, sink, refrigerator, microwave, and staff lockers |
| Staff toilet | 1 | 55 | 55 | Wheelchair accessible |
| **Subtotal (staff/administrative space)** | | | **415** | |
| **Total NSF** | | | **4,935** | Net square feet |
| Net-to-department gross factor | | × | 1.55 | |
| **Total DGSF** | | | **7,650** | Department gross square feet |

## ORGANIZING THE SPACE PROGRAM

The space program should be organized by major category of space to facilitate review by different constituencies, such as the following:

- *Patient intake space*, including reception, registration, patient and visitor waiting, and related amenities
- *Patient care, diagnostic, and treatment space*, such as inpatient rooms, exam rooms, procedure rooms, and treatment bays
- *Support space*, including clean and soiled utility rooms, medication rooms, and equipment storage areas that are neither used by patients nor occupied by staff on a full-time basis
- *Staff and administrative areas*, such as administrative offices and workstations, conference rooms, and staff lounges

For example, physician leaders will want to pay close attention to the patient care spaces and procedure rooms, while central registration, scheduling, and information systems staff will want to focus on patient intake space. Facilities management staff will need to review the number of procedure rooms that need to be equipped, and hospital leadership will want to review the staffing assumptions that drive the number of offices, workstations, and conference rooms.

## COMMON SPACES

Any space programming effort should begin with the identification of common spaces that can be replicated across departments or facility components in the healthcare facility. This standardization provides future flexibility and cost savings, as rooms serving comparable functions are similarly sized and finished instead of tailored to the individual occupants—even though the actual equipment and furnishings may be changed or upgraded over time. Larger healthcare organizations may already have developed a database of their own space standards and room layouts for frequently used rooms.

## KEY SPACE DRIVERS

A number of factors influence the type, size, and number of spaces in a given department or functional area. Key space drivers include the following:

- *Workload composition, patient mix, and scheduling patterns* primarily affect the type, number, and sizes of procedure rooms and patient preparation and recovery spaces.
- *Equipment and technology* affect the throughput of procedure rooms, which in turn affects the need for patient intake, waiting, preparation, and recovery spaces. Electronic management of information will affect the need for record storage space and will influence the flow of patients, staff, and materials throughout the department.
- *Staffing and scheduling* affect the number of staff offices and workstations needed as well as staff support facilities such as conference rooms, lockers, lounges, and toilet facilities.
- *Codes and regulations* affect the size of patient rooms, patient toilet and bathing facilities, specific procedures rooms, and other space described in the following sections.
- *The organization's mission and policies* may have a significant impact on the built environment at a healthcare center. Examples that often result in increased space allocation and construction costs include the following:
  - Decisions to invest in expansive lobbies and atriums to achieve an upscale (although sometimes ostentatious) image for the organization
  - Degree of commitment in the organization to optimizing the use of expensive diagnostic and treatment equipment—such as magnetic resonance imaging, computed tomography, and positron emission tomography—by promoting extended hours of operation
  - Inability to establish and enforce institution-wide space standards regarding office sizes by staff hierarchy, size and use of conference rooms, policies for staff lounges, and so on
  - Commitment to providing enhanced amenities for patients and visitors, such as comfortable lounges; dining areas; conference and education facilities; and other retail services such as gift shops, coffee shops, and an outpatient pharmacy
  - Commitment to providing enhanced amenities for physicians and employees, such as fitness centers, education and training facilities, and day care centers
  - Educational mission of the organization that requires classrooms, student lounges, and faculty offices
  - Research mission of the organization that requires space for clinical trials, offices for researchers, and dry and wet lab space

## ABOUT BUILDING CODES

The space program must comply with applicable building codes. The following codes vary by state or local municipality and should be reviewed and incorporated into the final space program:

- State hospital licensing rules
- State health agency codes
- State and local building codes
- State and local fire codes
- State and local handicap accessibility standards

Many building codes specify minimum sizes for traditional inpatient rooms, procedure rooms, and other related patient care spaces. The primary intent is to ensure public safety during the treatment or procedure, expedite egress for nonambulatory patients in case of a fire or other disasters, and provide accessibility for handicapped patients. Some examples of spaces for which minimum sizes are generally mandated include emergency department treatment cubicles, exam rooms, surgical operating rooms, labor and delivery rooms, recovery cubicles, patient toilet rooms, and private and multiple-bed inpatient rooms. The actual design and configuration of a specific room—for example, the direction of door swing or the length and width of room—and the equipment and furnishings may require minor adjustments to the space program during the design development stage.

In particular, the *Guidelines for Design and Construction of Hospitals and Outpatient Facilities* published by the Facilities Guidelines Institute (2014)—referred to as the FGI *Guidelines*—is used as either a code or a reference standard by The Joint Commission, many federal agencies, and authorities in 42 states when healthcare organizations review, approve, and finance projects. The *SpaceMed Guide* (Hayward 2015) complements the FGI *Guidelines* by helping healthcare providers, planners, and architects develop the functional and operational programs required prior to application of the FGI Guidelines, along with providing the room-by-room space requirements necessary to begin the design process.

## DEVELOPING SUPPLEMENTARY CONCEPTUAL DIAGRAMS

The operational and space program will often contain supplemental "bubble" diagrams that may be drawn to scale or may simply be conceptual in nature. The intent is to illustrate department workflow, physical space proximities and adjacencies, and other concepts to educate the task force members and to communicate the intent of the operational and space program to the design architect. Exhibit 8.2 presents an example of a conceptual diagram that may accompany the operational and space program.

## ENSURING AN EFFECTIVE PLANNING PROCESS

Historically, facility planning was often based on the wish lists of physicians and department managers. Unfortunately, some of the individuals who dominate the planning process move on to other organizations by the time the new or expanded facilities are ready for occupancy. Today, healthcare organizations realize that investments in facility expansion and reconfiguration must meet the needs of changing patient populations and providers during the life of the building. They cannot allow the planning process to be driven by the idiosyncrasies of a few individuals. Some healthcare organizations are challenging the more traditional bottom-up approach to operational and space planning and are choosing to embark on a more top-down approach, as shown in exhibit 8.3 (Hayward 2004).

---

**Exhibit 8.2 Example: Conceptual Diagram for an Emergency Department**

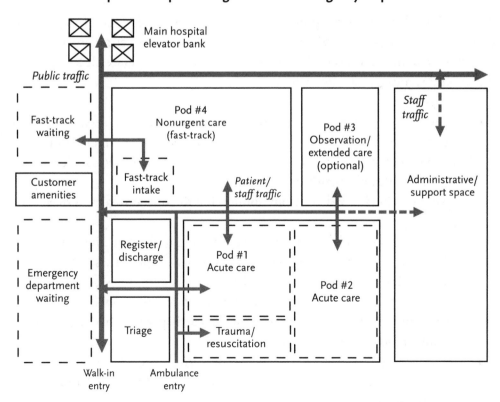

---

**Exhibit 8.3 Operational and Space Programming Approaches**

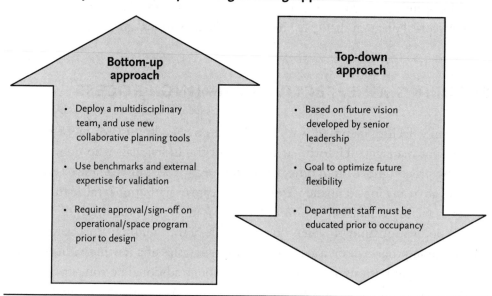

**Bottom-up approach**

- Deploy a multidisciplinary team, and use new collaborative planning tools

- Use benchmarks and external expertise for validation

- Require approval/sign-off on operational/space program prior to design

**Top-down approach**

- Based on future vision developed by senior leadership

- Goal to optimize future flexibility

- Department staff must be educated prior to occupancy

## Bottom-Up Approach

The traditional bottom-up approach involves the establishment of department user groups based on strict adherence to the organization's existing organizational structure. For the traditional bottom-up approach to be successful, healthcare organizations must do the following:

- Deploy a multidisciplinary team or task force to encourage department staff to think outside of their individual silos. Cross-departmental task forces, focused on common operational processes and patient needs, facilitate the planning of flexible healthcare space.
- Prevent specific individuals from dominating the operational and space planning process.
- Use some of the available collaborative planning tools to facilitate the gathering of input and the review of preliminary output. These methods allow multiple constituencies to participate in the process—for example, construct a project website that can accommodate online publishing of draft documents, around-the-clock review at the participants' convenience, and easy integration of their comments.
- Use industry benchmarks and external consulting expertise to validate internally generated space requirements and to introduce the planning team to new concepts and best practices.

- Consider site visits by selected task force members to peer institutions that have implemented unique operational models or have incorporated new technology as part of their facility planning efforts.
- Require approval of the operational and space program prior to commencing the schematic design stage. A formal process should be established for use by facility management and the design architect when changes are proposed to the space program during the schematic design and design development phases.

## Top-Down Approach

Some healthcare organizations prefer a more top-down approach, particularly when capital dollars are tight, when employee turnover at the department or service line manager level is high, or when market dynamics make program and workload forecasts difficult to discern. This approach is often used when hospital leadership is constructing a new or replacement healthcare facility, particularly when the leadership team wants to implement entirely new and innovative operational processes and technology. For this approach to be successful, healthcare organizations must do the following:

- Have a senior leadership team with a well-thought-out vision for the organization that can be communicated effectively.
- Bring in outside expertise to translate a future vision for the organization into flexible facilities that can accommodate future changes in medical practice and technology, accommodate various patient populations and providers, and facilitate quality and cost-effective patient care.
- Educate department staff about the vision and the new operational concepts and technology to be implemented prior to occupancy.

# PROGRAMMING INPATIENT NURSING UNITS

The planning of a large number of new or replacement beds requires a significant effort if your goal is an operationally efficient, patient-friendly, state-of-the-art facility. Of course, you can simply replicate your current operational concepts, level of technology, and staffing patterns with larger, newly furnished, private patient rooms. The operational and space programming process for constructing or replacing inpatient nursing units becomes somewhat more complicated than for most other hospital departments because of the magnitude of the impact of your decisions, such as labor costs and square feet. Exhibit 8.4 summarizes the many operational issues to be resolved when planning new inpatient nursing units. Resolving these issues generally requires a larger number of participants (or more task forces). Also, all task force members must be informed and educated about current best practices and must have the opportunity to make site visits to newly opened facilities and talk to their staff.

## RELATIONSHIP OF THE OPERATIONAL AND SPACE PROGRAM TO SUBSEQUENT DOCUMENTATION

The operational and space program should be coordinated with the equipment procurement plan and should be reviewed by appropriate central sources such as IT, materials management, admitting and registration, and other support departments. The workload projections and staffing assumptions can be incorporated into a financial feasibility analysis.

As the design architect proceeds with the design development phase (after approval of the schematic drawings), she will prepare *room data sheets* that correspond to each space delineated in the drawing and include detailed design information, such as floor and wall finishes; plumbing, electrical, and medical gas requirements; and similar information to be incorporated into the detailed construction documents.

When a department or service undergoes major expansion or reconfiguration or is relocated to new space, the operational and space program can provide the basis for subsequent development of an occupancy or building commissioning plan. Detailed occupancy planning generally begins as completion of the new facility approaches, and it includes items such as descriptions of new policies and procedures; revised job descriptions (as required); and a detailed schedule of tasks, dates, and responsibilities to ensure a smooth operational transition from the existing space to the new space. Because of the extended time frame from the preparation of the operational and space program through the design process to project construction and occupancy, the occupancy plan is generally developed separately from the predesign planning process and at a later date.

## TEN COMMON OPERATIONAL AND SPACE PROGRAMMING PITFALLS

An understanding of the predesign planning stage, terminology, and implementation of a formal operational and space programming process will prevent most

**Exhibit 8.4 Summary of Nursing Unit Operational Issues**

| Category | Operational Issues | Category | Operational Issues |
|---|---|---|---|
| Patient intake and processing | • Parking and wayfinding<br>• Admitting<br>• Patient transport (ancillary services, intra-unit transfers)<br>• Discharge (home, alternate facility)<br>• Consults (e.g., social services, pastoral care, infection control) | Patient and visitor amenities | • Television, DVD and music players<br>• Personal computing (e.g., Internet access, video games)<br>• Educational videos (live, recorded)<br>• Family and visitor lounge and sleeping facilities<br>• Consult and viewing areas |
| Communications | • Telephone (conventional, wireless)<br>• Personal computing (intranet and Internet)<br>• Nurse call or code blue<br>• Electronic tracking (staff, equipment, patients, visitors)<br>• Paging (overhead public address system, pocket pagers) | Network infrastructure | • Electronic health record<br>• Vital signs monitoring<br>• Picture archiving communication system<br>• Vendor neutral archive<br>• Video on demand<br>• Telemedicine (e.g., consultative, diagnostic, local area network, wide area network) |
| Clinical documentation | • Order entry<br>• Results reporting<br>• Consults<br>• Patient demographics<br>• Special forms<br>• Medication administration record<br>• Input and output<br>• Pain management<br>• Progress notes | Security | • Access control, surveillance, and detection<br>• Disaster planning and response (e.g., security, fire, earthquake, bioterrorism) |
| Clinical support | • Specimen collection, disposition, testing<br>• Medication delivery and dispensing (medication preparation rooms, self-contained automated medication-dispensing units or carts)<br>• Respiratory therapy (equipment monitoring, preparation, cleaning)<br>• Physical, occupational, and speech therapy<br>• Imaging | Materials management | • Materials and supply distribution (bar coding, scanning, self-contained automated supply cabinets)<br>• Food delivery (conventional, cook-freeze, cook-chill, convenience)<br>• Linen (clean delivery and soiled pickup)<br>• Environmental services<br>• Maintenance, engineering, biomedical<br>• Patient equipment and instrument processing<br>• Mail handling<br>• Trash, hazardous waste, recyclables<br>• Technology and communications equipment |

healthcare organizations from succumbing to the following common space planning pitfalls:

1. *Confusing net and gross space.* DGSF may be 25 percent to 50 percent higher than net square feet, and the building gross square feet may be another 25–35 percent higher than the DGSF.
2. *Planning additional procedure rooms, equipment, and expansion space for overly optimistic workload growth.* Because clinical departments typically plan staffing based on the number of procedure rooms, deploying an "if you build it, they will come" approach will result in increased labor and utility costs as well as higher up-front equipment costs.
3. *Planning offices and workstations for future staff members who have not been approved or for positions that will be eliminated.* This miscalculation will create pockets of vacant or underused space throughout the facility; however, the creation of flexible, generic office suites for use by multiple departments can mitigate this problem.
4. *Tailoring new facilities to the idiosyncrasies of a specific department manager or physician.* Current leadership may not be around when the new facility is opened, and the replacement leadership may want to instigate a new cycle of renovation projects.
5. *Failing to consider the staffing and other operational costs associated with larger, expanded facilities.* This tendency can be particularly problematic when revenues are flat.
6. *Replicating current, inefficient operational systems in new space.* It is more beneficial to rethink how patient care is delivered; evaluate ways to improve customer satisfaction; and identify opportunities to provide flexible, multiuse space.
7. *Focusing on space planning and the layout while ignoring the effect of interior design, furnishings, and cosmetic improvements.* Adequate dollars must be budgeted to enhance the look and feel of the space in addition to rectifying code noncompliances and resolving space deficiencies.
8. *Neglecting to consider the impact of new medical equipment and IT on procedure room throughput and required physical proximities.* Not considering these effects will result in overbuilding as well as increased operational costs and inefficient department layouts.
9. *Not planning for less efficient space use when retrofitting existing space for a new function.* This misstep will result in inappropriate and inadequate space for the planned functions. Older buildings are typically less flexible and have more unassignable space such as mechanical chases, numerous load-bearing

walls and partitions that can only be removed with great difficulty and at great expense, and fixed bay widths and column spacing.

10. *Beginning schematic drawings before an approved operational and space program is completed.* Failing to wait for the completed program will result in "scope creep," with the eventual size and cost of the project potentially escalating out of control.

## REFERENCES

Facilities Guidelines Institute (FGI). 2014. *Guidelines for Design and Construction of Hospitals and Outpatient Facilities*. Chicago: American Society for Healthcare Engineering of the American Hospital Association.

Hayward, C. 2015. *SpaceMed Guide: A Space Planning Guide for Healthcare Facilities*, 3rd ed. Ann Arbor, MI: HA Ventures.

———. 2004. "Rethinking Space Programming: Process, Approach, and Tools." Paper presented at the National Symposium on Healthcare Design, Las Vegas, Nevada.

# CHAPTER 9

# Case Study: Developing a Ten-Year Capital Investment Strategy for a Multihospital System

SOUTHERN HEALTH SYSTEM is a large not-for-profit healthcare system with more than 6,700 employees, 830 physicians on staff, and 928 licensed beds. At the time of the planning process, its three acute care campuses included the following:

1.  *General Hospital*, founded in 1920, was located about a mile south of the downtown area along a major north-south access road in a struggling commercial district. Its urban campus included a 427-bed hospital; a medical office center that housed physicians' offices; and the Rehabilitation Hospital, which had 60 inpatient beds and occupies the fifth and sixth floors. Numerous medical/surgical specialty services were provided, including a level II trauma center.

2.  *Suburban Hospital* opened in 2000 to serve the growing and affluent market south of the city, and it was designed with 220 beds. During the planning stage, the health system leadership decided to relocate the cardiac surgery program from General to Suburban and to offer high-risk obstetrics. The Children's Hospital operated 30 beds on the second floor of Suburban, including a pediatric intensive care unit (ICU), 40 neonatal intensive care beds (27 level II and 13 level III), a dedicated pediatric emergency department (ED), and a range of pediatric outpatient services.

3.  *Waterview Hospital* opened in 1985. It had served the residents of the surrounding communities for 30 years and was located across a waterway with access by toll bridge. The Waterview community was younger, less affluent, and somewhat isolated because of its geography. Initially constructed with 94 beds, Waterview had grown to 281 beds and provided general medical/surgical and specialty services, including high-risk

obstetrics. It was acquired by Southern Health in 2005 and maintained a separate medical staff.

Exhibit 9.1 illustrates the relative location and key characteristics of the three acute care campuses.

## 2015 CAPITAL INVESTMENT STRATEGY (FACILITY MASTER PLAN)

Southern Health conducted a comprehensive strategic planning process in late 2014 that identified the need for $155 million in capital investment across the three campuses, including $55 million for information technology (IT). In addition, the health system also considered a $22 million expansion project for the Children's Hospital at the Suburban site and an investment in a "medical mall" to be located across the street.

By 2015, the health system faced a number of major issues, including the following:

- *Diminishing operating margins.* Like many hospitals across the United States, Southern Health's operating margins had been declining.
- *Acute nursing shortage.* The region had an acute shortage of nursing staff, particularly during the peak winter season when premium wages are paid to traveling nurses.
- *Fluctuating market dynamics.* Organization leaders were concerned that Southern Health's high market share could diminish over time as new competitors focused on its growing market.
- *Licensed bed complement that did not reflect operational reality.* Compared with 928 total licensed beds, significantly fewer beds were needed, even during the peak winter season. Considering the most optimistic (high bed) scenario, Southern Health determined that it still would have a surplus of beds at the end of the decade. However, a significant portion of the licensed beds were at General, which was plagued by aging inpatient nursing units and lacked a sufficient number of private rooms and adequate support space to actually operate at the licensed capacity. At the same time, Suburban was at capacity and was concerned about its ability to accommodate current and future demand in its rapidly growing market.
- *Aging facilities at the flagship location.* Almost half of Southern Health's licensed beds were at General, where two-thirds of the total space was

**Exhibit 9.1 Southern Health's Existing Hospital Sites and Characteristics**

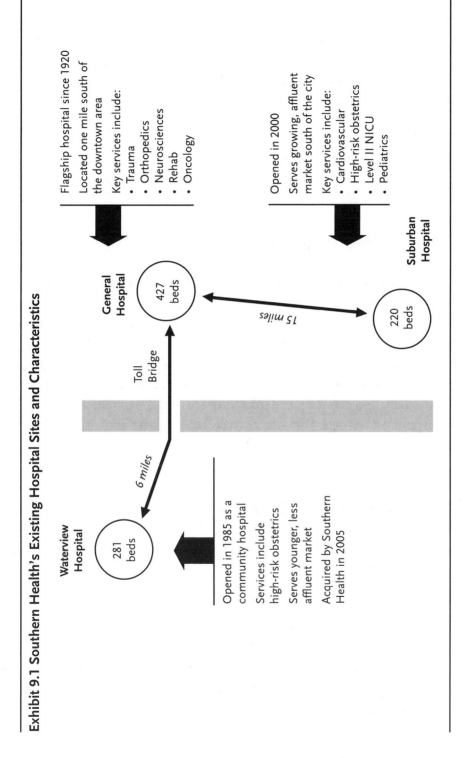

**Waterview Hospital**

281 beds

Opened in 1985 as a community hospital

Services include high-risk obstetrics

Serves younger, less affluent market

Acquired by Southern Health in 2005

**General Hospital**

427 beds

Flagship hospital since 1920

Located one mile south of the downtown area

Key services include:
- Trauma
- Orthopedics
- Neurosciences
- Rehab
- Oncology

**Suburban Hospital**

220 beds

Opened in 2000

Serves growing, affluent market south of the city

Key services include:
- Cardiovascular
- High-risk obstetrics
- Level II NICU
- Pediatrics

Toll Bridge

6 miles

15 miles

constructed prior to 1970. Moreover, ongoing capital investment had been minimal over the past decade. General was staffing 324 beds during its peak winter season. However, deployment of all of its 427 licensed beds was not possible. If all 427 beds were staffed, only 37 percent of the beds would be in private patient rooms, and 17 percent of the beds would need to be placed in three-bed and four-bed wards. In contrast, the 30-year old Waterview had been consistently maintained and upgraded, and the Suburban facility was only 15 years old. The Waterview and Suburban facilities were designed with only private patient rooms.

Southern Health decided that it needed a comprehensive facility master plan to guide capital investment over a ten-year period. The organization also wanted to reevaluate the alignment of key clinical services among its three acute care campuses.

## THE PLANNING PROCESS

The facility planning process included a review of historical utilization and market dynamics, identification of current facility assets and liabilities at the three acute care campuses, and an assessment of current and future space need by department and service line. The selected facility planning consultant led the development of a ten-year capital investment strategy based on projected future bed need and ancillary workloads and solicited input from department and service line leadership, the physician executive committee, and other physicians through individual interviews and focus group meetings. Periodic progress reports were made to the Southern Health executive council and the board.

## MAJOR FACILITY ASSETS AND LIABILITIES BY CAMPUS

An assessment of each campus resulted in an inventory of the facility assets and liabilities as shown in exhibit 9.2.

Key conclusions included the following:

- The General and Waterview facilities were underused.
- Although Suburban was at capacity, physician offices occupied more than 50,000 department gross square feet throughout the hospital that could be made available for other patient services if a new medical office building were constructed.

- Expansion of Suburban would require additional investment in the energy plant to increase its capacity.
- General has an aging physical plant that will require significant capital investment over time to maintain the status quo.

## MARKET DYNAMICS AND FUTURE BED NEED

In aggregate, Southern Health served an older but growing population. Its service area population was expected to grow by 20 percent through 2025, with 25 percent of the population older than 65. Although the highest growth rate was occurring in the southern portion of the county, Suburban's primary market, the highest growth in absolute numbers was occurring in Waterview's service area. The consensus was that Southern Health must protect its southern flank relative to cardiovascular surgery and general medical/surgical services. It was also agreed that the major competitive threat to the system's obstetrics services will come from the east.

Exhibit 9.3 summarizes Southern Health's bed complement. A detailed bed need analysis indicated that Southern Health needed approximately 500 acute medical/surgical beds (including the ICU) during its peak winter season and about 320 beds during the summer, compared to the 543 beds that were typically staffed. Use rates for the county were starting to decline, resulting in lower patient days despite a growing population. However, the health system consistently maintained an unusually high market share of about 67 percent.

The planning team projected that by 2025, Southern Health would still have a surplus of about 150 beds compared with the current licensed capacity, even in the high bed scenario, despite the significant population growth in the county. Because of fluctuating market dynamics and uncertainties, Southern Health leadership was reluctant to delicense beds at the time, particularly given the substantial growth to the south. Also, because Waterview served a market distinct from that of General, Southern Health leadership agreed that surplus beds at Waterview should not be delicensed until future population projections become evident.

## KEY FACILITY PRIORITIES

Several key facility investment priorities were identified that required action regardless of Southern Health's long-range facility investment strategy. These included the following:

**Exhibit 9.2 Southern Health's Major Facility Assets and Liabilities by Campus**

| Campus | Major Facility Assets | Major Facility Liabilities |
|---|---|---|
| General Hospital | • Located in the center of the community one mile south of the downtown area<br>• Level II trauma center designation<br>• 60-bed Rehabilitation Hospital<br>• Contiguous physician office building<br>• On-site wellness center<br>• Significant amount of vacant space available | • Site, parking, and wayfinding issues<br>• Outpatient services are fragmented<br>• General lack of public spaces and amenities<br>• Majority of medical/surgical beds are in older wings with limited private rooms and some older wards<br>• Separation of the medical/surgical ICUs creates staffing inefficiencies and limits flexibility<br>• Smith/Brown wings have severe code deficiencies |
| Suburban Hospital | • New facility with a high level of aesthetic appeal (e.g., large atrium)<br>• All inpatient beds in contemporary, private rooms<br>• Ample land for facility expansion<br>• High-profile cardiovascular service<br>• High-profile, NICU/obstetrics service with 36 LDRPs<br>• The Children's Hospital offers specialty pediatric services<br>• Contiguous physician office space | • Outpatient services are fragmented<br>• Multiple building entrances and intake points create further confusion<br>• Separation of surgical services on two different floors creates operational inefficiencies<br>• Energy plant will require upgrading to accommodate additional building expansion |
| Waterview Hospital | • Attached Women and Children's Pavilion with dedicated entrance and 23 LDRPs<br>• All inpatient beds in updated, private rooms<br>• Expansion space for surgery<br>• Contiguous physician office space<br>• Physical plant in excellent condition<br>• Vacant space available | • Multiple outpatient service locations with extensive walking distances, particularly from north to south<br>• Outpatient surgery prep/recovery area requires upgrading |

**Exhibit 9.3 Southern Health's Current Bed Complement**

|  | General | Suburban | Waterview | Total |
|---|---|---|---|---|
| Intensive care beds | 34 | 23 | 22 | 79 |
| Acute care beds | 215 | 91 | 158 | 464 |
| **Subtotal acute care (staffed)** | **249** | **114** | **180** | **543** |
| Rehab beds | 60 | — | — | 60 |
| LDRP beds | — | 36 | 23 | 59 |
| Pediatric beds | — | 30 | 9 | 39 |
| NICU bassinets | — | 40 | — | 40 |
| **Subtotal specialty beds (staffed)** | **60** | **106** | **32** | **198** |
| **Total staffed beds** | **309** | **220** | **212** | **741** |
| Vacant beds | 118 | — | 69 | 187 |
| **Current licensed beds** | **427** | **220** | **281** | **928** |

## General Hospital

- Reconfigure customer intake and outpatient services on the first floor to improve wayfinding, access, and convenience.
- Upgrade the surgery suite and invest in new equipment and technology to create a state-of-the-art facility.
- Combine the existing medical ICU (currently on the seventh floor) and the existing surgical ICU (currently on the eighth floor) to be on the second floor near the surgery suite to reduce staffing costs and enhance operational flexibility.
- Relocate the administrative services in the older Smith and Brown wings to the seventh and eighth floors to allow for demolition, thus avoiding further costly maintenance of these non–code compliant wings.

## Suburban Hospital

- Create an express testing area adjacent to the main entry in the space to be vacated by the community pediatric clinic.

- Immediately add unlicensed short-stay and observation beds to provide additional capacity—for example, an ED holding unit, pediatric observation unit, and adult short-stay beds.
- Expand or reconfigure surgical services and add a magnetic resonance imaging unit.

## Waterview Hospital

- Upgrade the ED and selected clinical services (noninvasive cardiology, sleep lab, and outpatient surgery recovery area).
- Convert a portion of the second floor to administrative offices and clinical support space.

# LONG-RANGE FACILITY DEVELOPMENT SCENARIOS

The facility planning consultant identified and evaluated three preliminary long-range facility development scenarios for the health system as follows.

## Scenario 1: Maintain the Status Quo

This scenario maintained the current distribution of beds and services among the three hospital campuses and assumed the conversion of three floors of General's north wing (no longer needed for inpatient space) to administrative services. The remaining five nursing units at General would be upgraded, and the number of private patient rooms would be increased.

## Scenario 2: Decompress Waterview Hospital

The intent of this scenario was to capitalize on the underused Women's and Children's Pavilion at Waterview by relocating high-risk obstetrics and the Children's Hospital from Suburban to Waterview. In this scenario, low-risk obstetrics would remain at Suburban, and the space occupied by pediatric services and the neonatal ICU (NICU) would be redeployed for additional medical/surgical bed capacity and the expanding cardiology program. The NICU would be expanded at Waterview, the underused second-floor nursing units would be redeployed for pediatrics, and physician offices on the first floor would be reassigned for obstetricians and pediatricians.

### Scenario 3: Decompress General Hospital

In this scenario, General would become a specialty center focused on orthopedics, neurosciences, and rehabilitation and would continue to maintain its trauma center status. Its bed complement would be reduced from the licensed capacity of 427 beds to approximately 172 beds (20 ICU, 72 acute care, 20 short-stay, and 60 rehabilitation). By substantially reducing the bed capacity at General, Southern Health would save significant money that had previously been slated for upgrading General's nine existing nursing units. The conversion of vacant inpatient space at General to office occupancy would allow the health system to consolidate various administrative services at General and discontinue the leasing of office space around the community.

## TEN-YEAR CAPITAL INVESTMENT STRATEGY FOR SOUTHERN HEALTH SYSTEM

The Southern Health executive council concluded that Scenario 1 was not feasible, because capital dollars were not available to maintain General at its current licensed bed capacity given the amount of renovation (and space) required to provide contemporary accommodations for 427 inpatients. Even maintaining its current staffed bed capacity would be difficult. At the same time, Suburban's inpatient census continued to rise, and there was concern that Southern Health was not positioned to compete aggressively for its share of the growing market south of the city (one of the fastest-growing areas in the United States).

Everyone agreed that Waterview had surplus capacity that could be readily used for obstetric and pediatric services—Suburban had 36 labor, delivery, recovery, and postpartum (LDRP) rooms and exceeded 3,000 annual births, while Waterview had 23 LDRP rooms and ample support space with only 900 annual births. However, getting the high-risk obstetricians and pediatric specialists to move their practices from Suburban to Waterview was not likely, at least not in the near future.

The executive council ultimately decided to pursue a variation of Scenario 3 that involved the transfer of 122 beds to Suburban by moving 81 medical/surgical beds from General and 41 beds from Waterview. Specific strategies, related actions, bed allocation, and capital needs were identified over the ten-year period, as illustrated in exhibit 9.4 and described in exhibit 9.5.

**Exhibit 9.4 Graphic Illustration of Southern Health's Ten-Year Capital Investment Strategy**

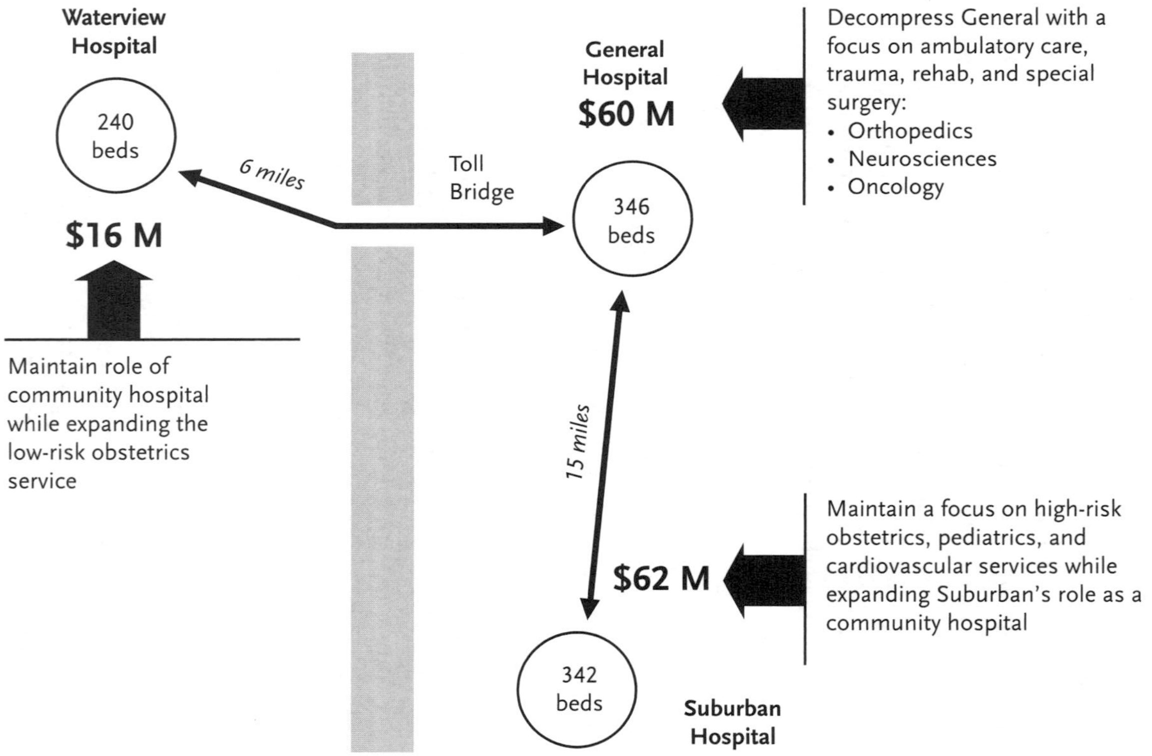

**Exhibit 9.5 Summary of Southern Health's Ten-Year Capital Investment Strategy**

| Campus | Immediate Strategy (Within Two Years) | Short-Term Strategy (Three to Five Years) | Long-Range Strategy (Five to Ten Years) |
|---|---|---|---|
| General Hospital | Improve patient intake/access and wayfinding and demolish oldest buildings:<br>• Create Customer Service Center<br>• Improve patient wayfinding and signage<br>• Demolish Smith Wing<br>• Add patient/visitor parking spaces<br>• Other general upgrading | Consolidate the medical and surgical ICUs, continue reconfiguring first and second floor clinical services, and convert surplus bed capacity to office occupancy:<br>• Upgrade the surgery suite<br>• Create consolidated ICU<br>• Reconfigure outpatient services (first floor)<br>• Convert 5/7/8-North to offices<br>• Other general upgrading | Decompress General with a focus on ambulatory care, trauma, rehab, and special surgery:<br>• Convert 4-MOC to neuro unit<br>• Upgrade ortho unit<br>• Convert 3-MOC to oncology unit<br>• Convert 6-North to offices<br>• Demolish Brown Wing<br>• Other general upgrading |
| Suburban Hospital | Address ED/bed capacity issues with specialty observation/short-stay units, and redirect low-risk obstetrics to Waterview:<br>• Create peds observation unit<br>• Create outpatient procedure unit<br>• Create short-stay unit<br>• Expand the ED<br>• Other general upgrading | Expand diagnostic/treatment services, improve outpatient intake/express testing, and increase medical/surgical bed capacity as census increases:<br>• Convert clinic to express testing<br>• Expand/reconfigure surgery suite<br>• Upgrade Energy Plant<br>• Add three floors (72–108 beds)<br>• Add patient/visitor parking spaces<br>• Other general upgrading | Maintain focus on high-risk obstetrics, pediatrics, and cardiovascular services while expanding Suburban's role as a community hospital |
| Waterview Hospital | Create office/staging space on 2-North and upgrade clinical services:<br>• Upgrade surgery post-op<br>• Convert 2-North to generic offices<br>• Upgrade the ED/other services<br>• Other general upgrading | Consolidate the clinical laboratory and upgrade/redeploy beds on second floor as census increases:<br>• Upgrade 2-East/West<br>• Consolidate laboratory<br>• Other general upgrading | Maintain role as a community hospital while expanding the low-risk obstetric service |

## DETAILED PROJECT PHASING AND IMPLEMENTATION PLAN

Southern Health's ten-year capital investment strategy was translated into distinct projects for which costs were estimated and time frames assigned. The ten-year capital investment plan for Southern Health will require approximately $138 million, excluding the cost of major equipment and IT, and will be allocated as follows:

- ◆ $38 million for immediate projects to be completed in two years
- ◆ $76 million for short-term projects to be completed in three to five years
- ◆ $24 million for long-term projects to be completed beyond five years

# CHAPTER 10

# Case Study: Planning an Ambulatory Care Facility

PRUDENT HEALTH SYSTEM planned to construct a new outpatient building on its main hospital campus to provide space for urgent care, ambulatory surgery, and various hospital-sponsored clinics. The organization needed space to accommodate the following ten-year workload projections and corresponding clinical services:

- Urgent care center with 32,000 annual visits
- Ambulatory surgery center with 4,200 annual surgical cases
- Hospital-sponsored clinics: medicine (23,000 annual visits), surgery (15,000 annual visits), neurosciences (6,000 annual visits), and orthopedics (16,000 annual visits)

In addition, Prudent Health planned a small express testing area to consolidate routine, quick-turnaround outpatient testing in a single area—including X-ray, electrocardiogram, and specimen collection—along with a small satellite laboratory.

A room-by-room space program was prepared on the basis of the projected workload and other functional planning assumptions provided by ambulatory care staff. The design architect developed an initial schematic drawing and the project cost was estimated. The Prudent Health staff then developed a business plan and a financial pro forma analysis.

Because of the large amount of space programmed and corresponding high project cost, as well as high operational costs relative to the projected incremental revenue, Prudent Health's chief financial officer asked the executive team whether it "really needed a Hummer when a compact Toyota might suffice." The executive team agreed to evaluate the impact on overall space need (and resulting capital and operational costs) of planning a lean facility.

## PLANNING APPROACH

The executive team reviewed the original operational assumptions documented in the functional program. In conjunction with the facility planning consultant, it identified several key factors that could reduce the overall size and cost of the new outpatient facility:

- *Operational assumptions.* Operational processes were reengineered to increase the exam and procedure room turnaround time. Weekly hours of operation were expanded, resulting in the need for fewer exam and procedure rooms. In addition to more efficient use of space, the changes would also enhance customer service.
- *Configuration of the clinics.* The clinics were originally programmed on the basis of their current organization and located in four distinct physical areas on the hospital campus. By combining the medicine, surgery, and neurology clinics into a single shared clinic, improved space use and staffing efficiencies would be possible. The new configuration also allowed the orthopedic clinic to be located on the first floor, thus eliminating one of the X-ray rooms and facilitating coverage by the radiology technicians working in the express testing area.
- *Size of exam and procedure rooms and offices.* Based on a review of its existing facilities, Prudent Health determined that it did not need such generously sized exam rooms and offices; for example, the clinic exam rooms were reprogrammed at 100 net square feet (NSF) versus 120 NSF, as originally programmed.
- *Facility design and layout.* Alternate facility layouts were chosen that resulted in less space required for intradepartmental and public circulation corridors. Along with two fewer floors, this change substantially reduced the amount of department gross square feet and building gross square feet (BGSF).

## COMPARISON OF FACILITY PLANNING ASSUMPTIONS AND SPACE NEED

The resulting space need is summarized in exhibit 10.1. In the lean scenario, 40,000 BGSF less space is required to accommodate the same projected annual workload. Exhibit 10.2 contains a summary of the assumptions used for the lean versus the more generous space planning approach.

**Exhibit 10.1 Comparison of Ambulatory Care Facility Space Need**

| | Space Program Summary | | |
|---|---|---|---|
| **Facility Component** | **Generous** | vs. | **Lean** |
| Urgent Care Center | 15,000 | | 8,600 |
| Ambulatory Care Center | 22,000 | | 13,100 |
| Orthopedics Clinic | 6,200 | | 3,700 |
| Medicine Clinic | 7,500 | | — |
| Surgery Clinic | 5,500 | | — |
| Neurology Clinic | 5,900 | | — |
| Shared Clinic | — | | 8,000 |
| Express Testing Area | 3,800 | | 3,400 |
| Entrance Lobby | 3,200 | | 3,200 |
| **Total DGSF** | **69,100** | | **40,000** |
| DGSF to BGSF conversion factor | 1.30 | | 1.25 |
| **Total BGSF** | **90,000** | vs. | **50,000** |

## CONCLUSION

With 40,000 BGSF less space required in the lean scenario to accommodate the same projected annual workload, the estimated project cost would be significantly reduced, particularly because the new space program required only two floors versus four, as originally planned (see exhibit 10.3). The Prudent Health executive team eventually decided to construct the smaller lean facility, which would also be less costly to operate over time than the more generous facility. Moreover, the cost savings allowed the facility to be designed to accommodate horizontal and vertical expansion in the future, as required.

# Exhibit 10.2 Comparison of Ambulatory Care Facility Planning Assumptions

| | Generous Space Program | Lean Space Program |
|---|---|---|
| Urgent Care Center<br>*32,000 annual visits* | • Staffed for limited weekly hours<br>• Average exam and treatment room turnaround time of 120 minutes<br>• Generously sized exam and treatment rooms and offices<br>• Private provider offices<br>• Generous NSF to DGSF space conversion factor | • Staffed for extended weekly hours<br>• Average exam and treatment room turnaround time of 75 minutes<br>• Moderately sized exam and treatment rooms and offices<br>• Shared provider offices<br>• Moderate NSF to DGSF space conversion factor |
| Ambulatory Surgery Center<br>*4,200 annual surgical cases* | • Staffed for limited weekly hours<br>• Average of 3.5 surgery cases per operating room per day<br>• Generously sized procedure rooms and prep/recovery bays<br>• Generous NSF to DGSF space conversion factor | • Staffed for extended weekly hours<br>• Average of 6.0 surgery cases per operating room per day<br>• Moderately sized procedure rooms and prep and recovery bays<br>• Moderate NSF to DGSF space conversion factor |
| Orthopedic Clinic<br>*16,000 annual visits* | • Staffed 48 weeks per year<br>• Average exam and treatment room turnaround time of 45 minutes<br>• Generously sized exam and treatment rooms and offices<br>• Dedicated X-ray room<br>• Private provider offices<br>• Generous NSF to DGSF space conversion factor | • Staffed 50 weeks per year<br>• Average exam and treatment room turnaround time of 40 minutes<br>• Moderately sized exam and treatment rooms and offices<br>• X-ray room shared with express testing area<br>• Shared provider offices<br>• Moderate NSF to DGSF space conversion factor |
| Other clinics:<br>Medicine Clinic<br>Surgery Clinic<br>Neurology Clinic<br>*44,000 annual visits* | • Staffed 48 weeks per year<br>• Three separate clinics with varying daily hours of operation and exam and treatment room turnaround times<br>• Four consult rooms and two larger testing and procedure rooms<br>• Generously sized exam and treatment rooms and offices<br>• Private provider offices<br>• Generous NSF to DGSF space conversion factor | • Staffed 50 weeks per year<br>• Shared clinic space with an average exam and treatment room turnaround time of 35 minutes<br>• Two consult rooms and one larger testing and procedure room (shared)<br>• Moderately sized exam and treatment rooms and offices<br>• Shared provider offices<br>• Moderate NSF to DGSF space conversion factor |

**Exhibit 10.3 Comparison of Ambulatory Care Facility Configuration Options (Building Section Diagram)**

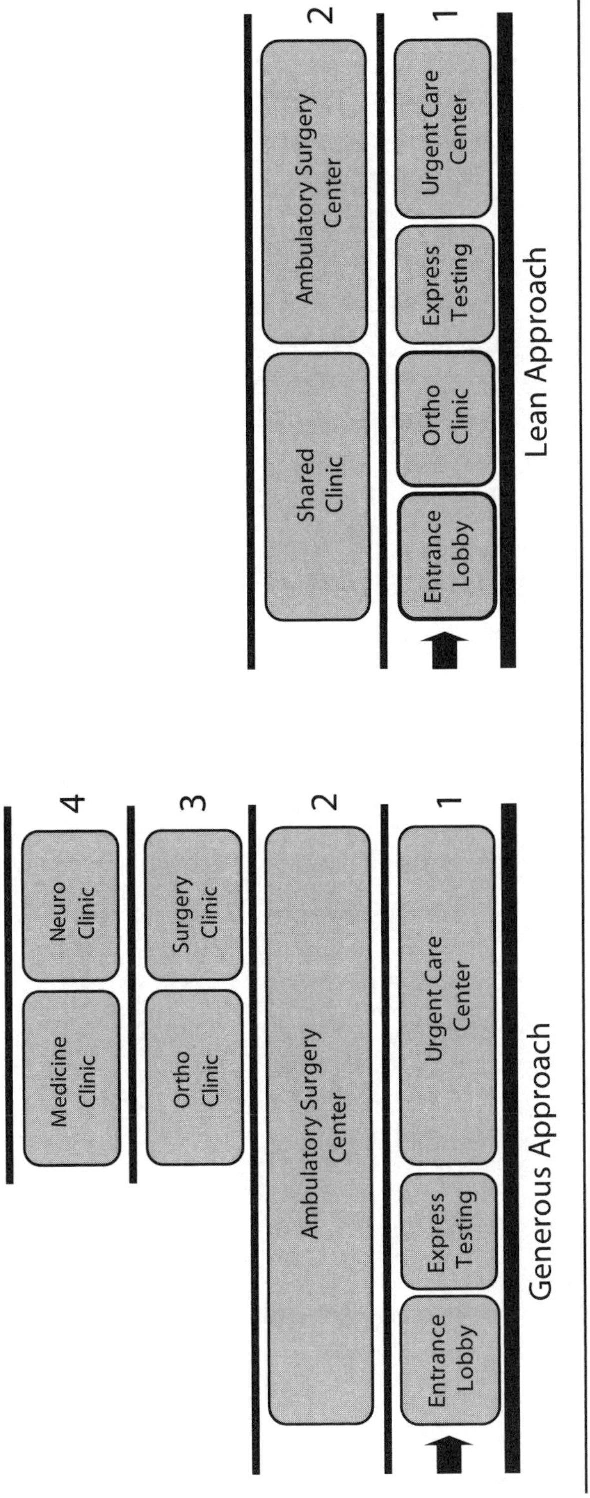

Generous Approach

| | | | |
|---|---|---|---|
| Medicine Clinic | Neuro Clinic | | 4 |
| Ortho Clinic | Surgery Clinic | | 3 |
| Ambulatory Surgery Center | | | 2 |
| Entrance Lobby | Express Testing | Urgent Care Center | 1 |

Lean Approach

| | | |
|---|---|---|
| Shared Clinic | Ambulatory Surgery Center | 2 |
| Entrance Lobby | Ortho Clinic / Express Testing / Urgent Care Center | 1 |

# CHAPTER 11

# Case Study: Evaluating Emergency Expansion

MIDWEST HOSPITAL PLANNED to expand and potentially replace its emergency department (ED) in response to increased crowding and congestion. Although the current number of annual visits (40,000) was not expected to grow significantly in the near future, the patient and visitor waiting room was frequently overflowing during the evening hours. ED staff also began creating "hall beds" by labeling and assigning defined stretcher bays in the hallways to gain additional treatment space during peak periods. Midwest viewed the relocation of an adjacent occupational medicine clinic as an option for ED expansion in lieu of total ED replacement.

Specific facility expansion goals included enlarging the patient and visitor waiting space and adding amenities; providing adequate exam and treatment space; triaging nonurgent patients in a separate, fast-track area; and developing a holding area for patients who are waiting for an available inpatient bed to be admitted. Although facility expansion and operations improvement were deemed necessary by all members of the planning team, the chief financial officer was concerned about spending significant capital dollars when ED revenues were relatively flat. ED staff also disagreed about the extent of required expansion; some wanted to almost double the size of the current ED, while others were concerned that significant expansion would require additional staff at a time when budgets were tight and recruiting was difficult. Others were concerned about the ED length of stay and its impact on customer satisfaction. However, all members of the planning team agreed that a detailed analysis of the relationship between improvements in exam and treatment room turnaround time and resulting space need and construction cost was warranted prior to initiating the detailed operational and space programming process.

# PLANNING APPROACH

The ED leadership assembled a detailed database and identified a number of operational issues that would ultimately affect the size of the upgraded ED:

- *Trends in ED utilization and patient mix.* Historically, emergency visits at Midwest increased 2–4 percent annually; however, ED visits had stabilized at around 40,000 annually during the past two years. The leveling off had been generally attributed to a community-wide initiative to redirect the uninsured to primary care clinics. However, Midwest's ED had been on diversion frequently because of a lack of intensive care beds at the hospital. Both the percentage of ED patients who were admitted (currently at 18 percent) and the percentage of nonurgent care patients (currently at 40 percent) had been increasing, even though total ED volume had stabilized.
- *Treatment room turnaround time.* The average treatment room turnaround time at Midwest was more than three hours, which is even longer when the time from initial triage to placement in the treatment room and the time from exiting the treatment room to eventual discharge were added. Critical operational issues included slow responsiveness from the imaging department for magnetic resonance imaging scans and long waiting times for physician consultations. The backup of patients to be admitted while they were waiting for an available inpatient bed was also a major issue.
- *Number of treatment bays.* A total of 30 ED treatment spaces were available, including two large triage and resuscitation rooms and dedicated rooms for obstetrics/gynecology and orthopedic casting. Four of the treatment bays were designated for nonurgent patients, although they were generally used on a first-come-first-served basis with no formal fast-track process in place. In addition, dedicated X-ray and computed tomography rooms were located in the ED.
- *Average net square feet (NSF) per treatment bay.* The existing treatment rooms and bays average only 105 NSF, with some stretcher bays sized at less than 70 NSF (contemporary standards are 120 NSF for general ED treatment rooms, increasing to more than double the space for trauma and resuscitation rooms).
- *Ratio of total department gross square feet (DGSF) per treatment room to bays.* The ratio of the current amount of DGSF to the total number of treatment and procedure rooms (or bays) was evaluated to assess the adequacy of the overall footprint of the ED to support the current number of treatment rooms and bays. With 11,250 DGSF occupied by the current ED, the current average was only 375 DGSF per treatment space (contemporary

design standards are 550–650 DGSF per treatment or procedure space). This result confirmed a severe shortage of support space and inadequately sized treatment cubicles.

◆ *Average annual visits per treatment bay.* With 40,000 annual ED visits and 30 treatment bays and rooms, Midwest accommodated 1,333 annual ED visits per treatment room or bay.

## EFFECT OF TREATMENT ROOM TURNAROUND TIME ON EMERGENCY DEPARTMENT SPACE AND PROJECT COSTS

The ED leadership then analyzed the impact of treatment room turnaround time on required ED treatment rooms, total DGSF, and total project cost. The analysis revealed that even minor improvements in ED turnaround time would have a significant effect on the space and resulting renovation or construction costs, as shown in exhibit 11.1.

## CONCLUSION

Because of the high cost of replacing the existing ED, particularly if 30 or more treatment cubicles and support space were provided, the ED planning team ultimately decided to focus its operations improvement efforts on improving ED treatment room turnaround time, with a target of 120 minutes, before embarking on a major renovation or construction project.

Because the adjacent occupational health clinic (with six exam rooms and support space) scheduled patients only from Monday through Friday and was typically

**Exhibit 11.1 Impact of Treatment Room Turnaround Time on ED Space and Project Costs (Assuming 40,000 Annual Visits)**

| Average Treatment Bay Turnaround Time | Treatment Bays Required | Gross Space Required at 550 to 650 DGSF per Bay | Estimated Project Cost |
|---|---|---|---|
| 90 minutes | 20 | 11,000–13,000 | $4.7–$5.5 million |
| 120 minutes | 25 | 13,750–16,250 | $5.8–$6.9 million |
| 180 minutes | 35 | 19,250–22,750 | $8.2–$9.7 million |

closed at 4:00 pm each day, and because ED demand for nonurgent (fast-track) space typically occurred between 4:00 pm and 11:00 pm, ED leadership developed an operational plan to use the occupational health clinic's space to triage and treat nonurgent ED patients during the evenings and weekends. With the diversion of these nonurgent patients out of the main ED, the smallest ED treatment rooms and bays were reconfigured, resulting in 25 appropriately sized ED treatment rooms and cubicles in addition to the six fast-track exam and treatment rooms. The ED undertook a modest expansion of the patient and family waiting area using adjacent office space. This interim solution allowed Midwest to monitor trends in ED volume and evaluate the success of its operations improvement efforts. Hospital leadership agreed to reevaluate the need for a major ED expansion or replacement project in another year.

# CHAPTER 12

# Case Study: Developing a Bed Expansion Plan

COMMUNITY HOSPITAL WAS originally designed to accommodate 250 licensed beds with only 60 percent of the beds in private patient rooms (150 beds). The remaining 100 beds were located in semiprivate rooms, resulting in a total of 200 actual rooms (150 privates and 50 semiprivates). The average daily census was 205 inpatients, resulting in an average occupancy of 82 percent. The mix of private and semiprivate rooms, however, was misleading because Community rarely placed more than one patient per room in the oldest nursing units. Because of concerns with patient privacy, infection control, and medical errors, along with undersized semiprivate patient rooms, Community leadership wanted to develop a bed expansion and replacement plan to address inpatient demand through the next ten years.

Although some bed replacement and expansion were deemed necessary by all members of the planning team, the chief financial officer (CFO) was concerned about spending significant capital dollars given current economic conditions. Community executives also did not agree on the extent of the required expansion—some wanted to plan for 100 percent private rooms, while others were concerned that significant expansion would require additional staff at a time when recruiting was difficult and budgets were tight. Others were concerned about losing admissions to competitor hospitals who had more contemporary patient accommodations. Declining length of stay (LOS) was also a concern. However, everyone agreed that the current use rate (admissions per 1,000 population) would most likely remain constant. They also agreed that the county's updated ten-year population forecast was reasonable, given that it was much lower than previous estimates.

## PLANNING APPROACH

The Community executive team was not interested in projecting the need for an absolute number of beds at some future date. Instead, Community wanted to identify the range of beds required, on the basis of the most optimistic and pessimistic views of future market conditions—particularly because decisions to expand or replace its inpatient facilities would start a chain reaction and involve a long-range commitment of dollars, staff time, and operational disruption.

All members of the planning team agreed that a sensitivity analysis was needed to model the impact of different planning assumptions on future bed need and to evaluate the magnitude of renovation or construction. They also wanted to look at the relationship between high bed need and low bed need scenarios and the resulting number of private patient rooms that could be available.

As shown in exhibit 12.1, different scenarios were modeled based on varying market share, LOS, and occupancy rate assumptions, with the use rate and projected service area population held constant as follows:

- *Population.* A population increase of 9 percent was projected in all scenarios. The medium bed need scenario reflects the status quo relative to all other variables.
- *Use rate.* The use rate was projected to remain constant in all scenarios at 110.5 admissions per 1,000 population in Community's service area.
- *Hospital market share.* Community's market share was projected to decrease by 5 percent in the low bed need scenario and increase by 10 percent in the high bed need scenario.
- *Hospital admissions.* Community's admissions were calculated by applying the use rate to the projected service area population and multiplying by the hospital's expected market share.
- *Average LOS.* Community's current average LOS was reduced by one half-day in the low bed need scenario and maintained in the high bed need scenario.
- *Average daily census.* The expected average daily patient census for Community was calculated by multiplying the projected admissions by the LOS and dividing by 365 days.
- *Bed need.* Community's projected ten-year bed need was calculated based on varying occupancy levels.

The target occupancy rate was also an issue for Community. The hospital typically used 80 percent occupancy as a target. However, Community realized that organizations with only private patient rooms are reevaluating this target. Given planning

# Exhibit 12.1 Comparison of Future Bed Need Scenarios

| | Today | Ten-Year Bed Need Scenarios | | |
| --- | --- | --- | --- | --- |
| | | Low Bed Need (Declining Market Share and LOS) | Medium Bed Need (Status Quo with Population Increase Only) | High Bed Need (Increased Market Share Only) |
| Service area population | 445,030 | 485,000 | 485,000 | 485,000 |
| Use rate (admissions/1,000) | 110.5 | 110.5 | 110.5 | 110.5 |
| Hospital market share | 27.6% | 26.2% | 27.6% | 30.4% |
| Hospital admissions | 13,573 | 14,041 | 14,792 | 16,292 |
| Length of stay (LOS) | 5.50 | 5.00 | 5.50 | 5.50 |
| Average daily census | 205 | 192 | 223 | 245 |
| Bed need at: | | | | |
| 90% occupancy | | 214 | 248 | 273 |
| 85% occupancy | | 226 | 262 | 289 |
| 80% occupancy | | 240 | 279 | 307 |
| Current bed capacity | 250 | 250 | 250 | 250 |
| Bed surplus (+) or deficit (−) | | +36 to +10 | +2 to −29 | −23 to −57 |

uncertainties and the high cost of construction, Community's CFO was willing to accept the risk of not accommodating all demand during peak periods to avoid having vacant patient rooms during average census periods. The planning director noted that, statistically, a hospital with all private patient rooms should be able to maintain a higher occupancy level than one with a large number of semiprivate or multiple-bed rooms. On the other hand, targeting a higher occupancy level would not be practical for Community if it maintained its current high percentage of semiprivate patient rooms. The hospital decided to use a target of 85 percent occupancy, assuming that it needed to increase the number of private patient rooms regardless.

The Community leadership team had the following observations regarding the ten-year bed need projections:

- The 9 percent increase in population alone (all scenarios) resulted in the need for an additional 12 beds (total of 262 beds at 85 percent occupancy).
- In the high bed need scenario, a 10 percent increase in market share resulted in the need for an additional 39 beds (total of 289 beds at 85 percent occupancy).
- In the low bed need scenario, with both the market share and LOS reduced, 24 fewer beds would be needed (total of 226 beds at 85 percent occupancy).
- Assuming a lower occupancy target of 80 percent resulted in the need for 14–18 more beds depending on the scenario; assuming a higher occupancy rate of 90 percent resulted in a reduction of 12–16 beds.

## ANALYSIS

Exhibit 12.2 displays the high bed need and low bed need scenarios projected through the next ten years with varying occupancy assumptions. The hospital's current licensed capacity of 250 beds is also shown, along with the existing number of patient rooms—regardless of whether some were originally designed to accommodate two patients.

### Low Bed Need Scenario

Because this facility was originally designed with a total of 200 patient rooms (150 privates and 50 semiprivates), in the low bed need scenario Community could essentially use all the patient rooms as privates during the average daily census (192 patients) while retaining a limited number of semiprivate rooms to accommodate

**Exhibit 12.2 Impact of Varying Occupancy Rates on Bed Need Scenarios**

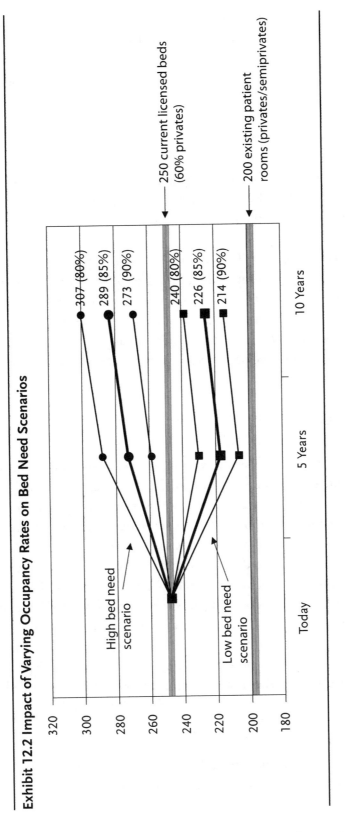

307 (80%)
289 (85%)
273 (90%)
240 (80%)
226 (85%)
214 (90%)

250 current licensed beds (60% privates)

200 existing patient rooms (privates/semiprivates)

High bed need scenario

Low bed need scenario

Today

5 Years

10 Years

320
300
280
260
240
220
200
180

peak census periods and maintain its current licensure. No expansion would be necessary for ten years unless Community desired to upgrade or replace some of the existing patient rooms—such as enlarging the patient rooms and providing wheelchair-accessible toilet and bathing facilities as well as additional amenities.

### High Bed Need Scenario

Bed expansion would definitely be required in the high bed need scenario to accommodate the ten-year bed need. If the high bed need scenario comes to fruition, Community considered the following possible bed-expansion strategies:

- *Conservative approach.* Construct 40 additional private patient rooms, thus increasing the proportion of private patient rooms to 66 percent; Community would only need to put two patients in the semiprivate rooms when the average daily census exceeds about 83 percent.
- *Aggressive approach.* Construct 90 additional private patient rooms, resulting in 100 percent of the projected beds in private rooms in ten years.

## CONCLUSION

The Community executive team recognized that even though the low bed need scenario resulted in fewer beds than were then licensed, Community was effectively using 220 beds rather than 250. Some of the semiprivate patient rooms in the two oldest nursing units were too small to accommodate two patients, given the amount of equipment and technology used today to deliver inpatient care. The team decided that even in the low bed need scenario, the hospital still needed to replace at least 30 beds. This change would result in a total of 230 patient rooms that could all be used as privates if the low bed need scenario occurs—assuming that the resulting number of beds per nursing unit did not compromise staffing efficiencies.

The Community executive team agreed on the goal of enough patient rooms to accommodate the ten-year projected average daily census of 245 patients (high bed need scenario). Some of the existing semiprivate patient rooms would be maintained and deployed during high census periods if the high bed need scenario evolves.

Ultimately, Community developed a plan to construct 72 new beds, all in private rooms. Approximately 20 semiprivate patient rooms would be maintained to accommodate peak census periods. Depending on the future bed need, the two oldest nursing units could be redeployed for same-day and observation patients, although the beds could still be used as overflow inpatient beds at some point if necessary. With the existing 150 private patient rooms, 30 converted private rooms (existing semiprivates), 72 new private patient rooms, and 20 remaining semiprivate patient rooms, Community could expand its licensure to 292 beds to accommodate the high bed need scenario for the ten-year planning horizon. If this scenario does not come to fruition, the oldest nursing units could be permanently decommissioned for an alternative use and all of the remaining semiprivate patient rooms could be converted for single-patient use. This plan would result in a total of 242 private patient rooms.

Like many hospitals, Community was challenged with planning a staged conversion of semiprivate patient rooms to privates over time while maintaining sufficient flexibility to offset forecasting inaccuracies. If the low bed need scenario played out, then some of the existing semiprivate patient rooms could be used for single occupancy. On the other hand, if the high bed need scenario evolved, then Community would need to deploy some of the rooms as semiprivates during peak census periods.

# CHAPTER 13

# Case Study: Consolidating
# Two Acute Care Hospitals

OCEAN HEALTH SYSTEM included three acute care hospitals, with a total capacity for 670 beds, although each hospital staffed significantly fewer beds:

- Valley Hospital with 245 beds
- Coast Hospital with 360 beds
- Rural Hospital with 65 beds

Valley and Coast were located six miles apart in a scenic northeastern region. Acute care beds were located at both sites, along with duplicative emergency departments (EDs), surgical suites, and various diagnostic and support services. Both of these facilities shared essentially the same market, along with a competitor hospital to the northeast.

Rural, although only eight miles away from Valley, required travel via a congested and winding road, with travel time averaging 20–30 minutes. Rural also had a distinctly different patient catchment area from Valley and Coast. Most Rural patients came from the west, where it competed with hospitals bordering a large urban area.

## KEY PLANNING ISSUES

Ocean Health contracted with a facility planning consultant to help its leadership develop a clinical service realignment plan based on an evaluation of key clinical and support services, current resources (staffing, equipment, space, and facilities), patient origin, and other market characteristics. The goal was to eliminate systemwide redundancies and minimize operational costs while maintaining or increasing market share. Because Rural served a distinctly different market from the Coast and Valley markets, consolidation of Rural with the other two acute care facilities would negatively affect market share. Therefore, Ocean Health decided to maintain the status quo as to Rural's geographic location and current array of services—acute medical/surgical beds, a full-service ED, inpatient and outpatient surgery, diagnostic radiology, computed tomography (CT), nuclear medicine, and noninvasive cardiac diagnostics.

## PROPOSED FACILITY CONSOLIDATION PLAN

As illustrated in exhibit 13.1, Ocean Health planned a new 210-bed hospital with a community hospital focus and centers of excellence in obstetrics, cardiology, and cancer care. The Valley site would continue to be used for inpatient subacute, rehabilitation, and psychiatric services, along with outpatient dialysis, physical and occupational therapy, and psychiatry. The older wings would be demolished to reduce the overall space to be maintained at this site. Rural would be maintained with a community hospital and short-stay focus, and Coast would be demolished and the land sold off to a local developer for an alternate use. Exhibit 13.2 displays the proposed clinical service realignment plan.

As shown in exhibit 13.3, the organization's leadership anticipated a reduction in the need for expensive procedure rooms or treatment spaces—and corresponding equipment and staffing—with the consolidation of the Valley and Coast acute care services into a single new, efficient facility. The elimination of six emergency treatment bays, three diagnostic radiology rooms, one CT scanner, one nuclear medicine camera, and two operating rooms—to accommodate the same or a greater number of procedures—had significant cost implications for both the initial capital cost of new construction and long-term operational costs.

## COMPARISON OF EXISTING AND NEW SPACE

The construction of a new, efficient facility resulted in significant space reduction, as shown in exhibit 13.4.

Prior to construction of the new facility, Coast and Valley together used 532,000 building gross square feet (BGSF). The new facility would require only 340,000 BGSF, with 80,000 remaining at the existing Valley site to accommodate postacute,

**Exhibit 13.1 Proposed Facility Consolidation Plan**

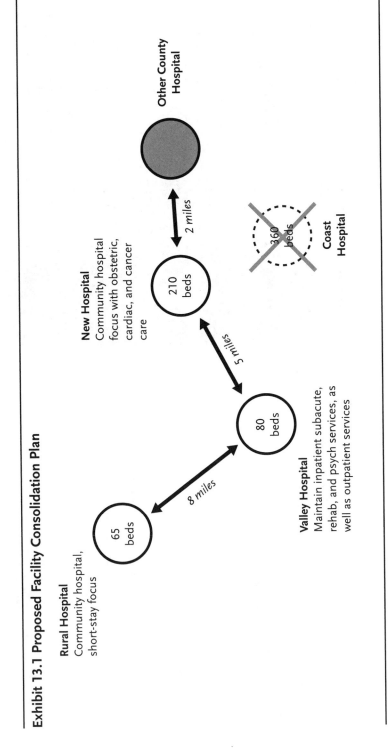

**Rural Hospital**
Community hospital, short-stay focus

65 beds

8 miles

80 beds

**Valley Hospital**
Maintain inpatient subacute, rehab, and psych services, as well as outpatient services

5 miles

210 beds

**New Hospital**
Community hospital focus with obstetric, cardiac, and cancer care

2 miles

Other County Hospital

360 beds

**Coast Hospital**

**Exhibit 13.2 Proposed Clinical Service Realignment Plan**

| | Clinical Service | Coast Hospital Site | Valley Hospital Site | New Hospital Site | Rural Hospital Site |
|---|---|---|---|---|---|
| Inpatient services | Acute medical/surgical | Closed | No | Yes | Yes |
| | Subacute | Closed | Yes | No | No |
| | Rehabilitation | Closed | Yes | No | No |
| | Psychiatry | Closed | Yes | No | No |
| | Obstetrics | Closed | No | Yes | No |
| Outpatient servcices | Emergency | Closed | No | Yes | Yes |
| | Surgery | Closed | No | Yes | Yes |
| | Imaging/special procedures | Closed | No | Yes | Yes |
| | Cardiac rehabilitation | Closed | No | Yes | Yes |
| | Dialysis | Closed | Yes | No | Yes |
| | Physical/occupational therapy | Closed | Yes | No | Yes |
| | Psychiatry | Closed | Yes | No | No |
| | Radiation therapy | Closed | No | Yes | No |

rehabilitation, and psychiatric services. With Coast closed, a total of 420,000 BGSF would be needed to accommodate the same or higher workloads compared to the existing 532,000 BGSF. This consolidation resulted in a savings of 112,000 BGSF (a 21 percent reduction).

**Exhibit 13.3 Comparison of Existing and New Treatment Spaces**

| | Current Procedure Rooms/Bays | | | | |
| Modality | Coast Hospital | Valley Hospital | Total | Combined Need | Variance |
| --- | --- | --- | --- | --- | --- |
| Emergency Treatment | 10 | 14 | 24 | 18 | (6) |
| Diagnostic Imaging | 4 | 4 | 8 | 5 | (3) |
| Computed Tomography | 1 | 1 | 2 | 1 | (1) |
| Nuclear Medicine | 1 | 2 | 3 | 2 | (1) |
| Surgery | 4 | 5 | 9 | 7 | (2) |

**Exhibit 13.4 Comparison of Existing and New Space**

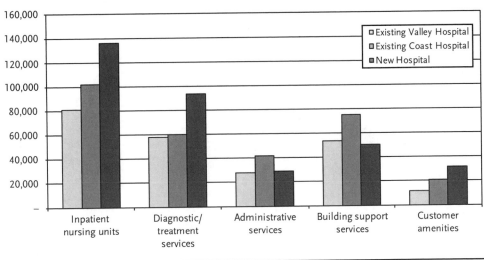

# CHAPTER 14

# Case Study: Planning a Prototype Community Health Center

NORTHERN HEALTH AUTHORITY delivers healthcare to the residents of 20 different communities that are a mix of settlements, towns, and villages. With many of its existing remote community health centers in need of replacement, Northern Health decided to develop a prototype community health center that could be replicated to serve communities of less than 1,500 people—some of which are accessible only by air.

## THE CHALLENGE

The challenge was to develop a community-oriented, culturally sensitive facility focused on wellness to reflect Northern Health's new integrated service delivery model. This client-centered approach to providing health and social services focused on illness prevention and health promotion using a multidisciplinary team of nurses, social workers, mental health and addiction counselors, and other community-based and visiting staff. At the same time, Northern Health needed to provide operational flexibility with generic, multiuse, technically adaptable spaces to allow visiting and rotating staff to function efficiently regardless of the facility they were assigned to.

Northern Health contracted with a facility planning consultant to first prepare operational plans for small, medium, and large community health centers based on a demand analysis and an assessment of the existing community health centers. The facility planning consultant then developed a space planning methodology and facility configuration concept that could be scaled up or down on the basis of the assigned staff and availability of local and regional services. This flexibility would allow a detailed operational and space program to be easily prepared for each new community health center as it is replaced.

To optimize the work flow and circulation and to minimize construction costs, the facility planning consultant undertook a structured planning process that identified generic spaces to be located in the community health center, determined the factors that drive the size and number of individual spaces required, and aggregated space by its function.

## FACILITY PLANNING PRINCIPLES

After a review of the planned scope of services, hours of operation, projected staffing, and support service assumptions documented in the operational plan, key facility planning principles were established:

◆ The community health center should be community oriented and culturally sensitive, and it should focus on wellness.
◆ The community health center environment should be safe and secure.
◆ Advanced technology should be embraced to the fullest extent possible.
◆ Spaces should be multifunctional, flexible, and adaptable as programs, services, and technology evolve over time.
◆ All community health centers should be configured similarly to allow staff to easily work in any facility with minimal orientation.

## IDENTIFYING GENERIC SPACES

After all potential spaces were identified, standardized room layouts and data and specification sheets were developed for generic spaces that accommodated similar functions and could be replicated in each community health center. This approach provided both flexibility and savings because rooms would be similarly sized and finished, not tailored to the occupants at a particular site.

## DETERMINING KEY SPACE DRIVERS

A specific space driver was determined for each individual room or area to be located in the prototype community health center (illustrated in exhibit 14.1):

- *Staffing-dependent.* The number of exam and treatment rooms, offices, consultation rooms, and administrative workstations were based on the expected daily head count—including nurses, social workers, mental health and addiction counselors, and support staff.
- *Variable.* The number of waiting room seats and client toilet rooms will vary on the basis of the total number of exam, treatment, or consult rooms in which clients will be routinely scheduled during the day. At the same time, the size of the mechanical room depended on the overall size of the facility.
- *Fixed.* All other spaces would generally not vary in either number or size, regardless of the overall scope of activities and projected staffing at a specific community health center.
- *Optional.* In addition, the decision to include on-site provider apartments versus a single staff sleep room in the community health center would depend on housing availability in a specific community.

**Exhibit 14.1 Key Space Drivers for the Prototype Community Health Center**

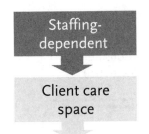

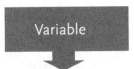

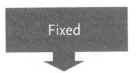

Staffing-dependent

Variable
- Waiting seats
- Client toilet rooms
- Mechanical room

Fixed
- Entry vestibules
- Group meeting room
- Emergency treatment room
- Multipurpose screening room
- Medication room
- Laboratory
- Clean/soiled utility rooms
- Kitchen/dining room
- Laundry room
- General storage room
- Housekeeping room
- Other

Client care space
- Exam/treatment rooms
- Office/consult rooms
- Dental treatment room

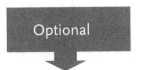

Optional
- On-site provider apartments
- Staff sleep room

Administrative space
- Reception office
- Private offices
- Workstations/cubicles

# ORGANIZING SPACE INTO FUNCTIONAL CATEGORIES

The space planning guidelines for the prototype community health center were organized into five major categories of space relating to specific activity zones in the prototype facility:

1. *The public reception zone* included the main entrance to the community health center and associated public spaces and amenities.
2. *The client care zone* comprised spaces for client assessment, treatment, and counseling along with associated support space.
3. *The staff administrative zone* was for the exclusive use of the staff assigned to the community health center.
4. *The building support zone* included housekeeping, storage, mechanical, and other spaces that supported the facility but were not routinely occupied by staff.
5. *The provider housing* was located on-site and included four one-bedroom apartments with a shared entrance and laundry room.

**Exhibit 14.2 Prototype Community Health Center Activity Zones**

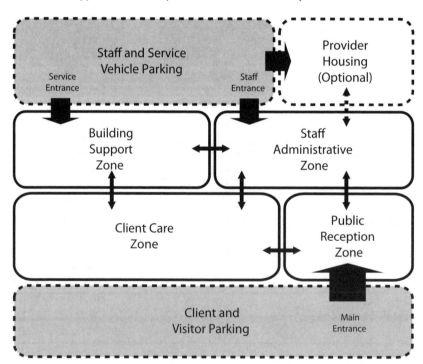

As illustrated in exhibit 14.2, clients and visitors would arrive at the community health center, park as necessary, and enter the building via the main entrance leading directly into the public reception zone. From this area, clients would be escorted to the client care zone when the provider was ready. Access to the staff administrative and building support zones would be for the exclusive use of the staff and secured from public access. Dedicated service and staff entrances would not be visible from the main entrance (e.g., at the rear of the facility), to avoid confusion.

## FUTURE EXPANSION

The community health center was designed to accommodate future expansion if required. The organization of the facility into distinct "zones" would facilitate the expansion of one or more specific zones—independent of the others—although demand for additional client care and staff administrative space would be greatest.

Because of the economies of scale, the planned building support spaces have the capacity to accommodate significant future growth in client activity volume. Likewise, the public reception zone does not necessarily need to expand in proportion to the client care zone, depending on whether throughput was improved, hours of operation were extended, and other factors. The provider housing could also be expanded independently of the community health center itself.

## CONCLUSION

By developing a space planning methodology—and a generic space programming template and a conceptual facility layout—the process of preparing an operational and space program and schematic design for each new Northern Health community health center could be expedited. In addition, this approach would result in short-term operational efficiencies and long-term operational flexibility while minimizing construction and renovation costs.

# CHAPTER 15

# Optimizing Current and Future Flexibility

The term *flexibility* has become somewhat overused today. It is repeated as a mantra among healthcare planners and design architects. By definition, it means adaptable or adjustable to change. In reality, achieving flexibility often requires that physicians, department managers, and staff relinquish absolute control over their space and equipment for the greater good of the organization (Hayward 2015).

## WHY IS FLEXIBILITY IMPORTANT?

Many of the reasons that we need to provide flexible and adaptable healthcare facilities have already been addressed in previous chapters of this book. Some of these reasons include the following:

- The unpredictable healthcare environment, with fluctuating demand driven by changing reimbursement, new regulations, and media attention to specific procedures and treatments
- The blending and melding of many diagnostic and treatment modalities as a result of advances in technology
- Staffing shortages in many specialties that necessitate the cross-training of staff and the creation of new job descriptions
- Electronic information management that eliminates the need for physical proximity
- Limited access to capital that requires ever more efficient use of all resources, including staff, equipment, and space

# DIFFERENT WAYS OF ACHIEVING FLEXIBILITY

Facilities should be planned to *optimize current space* as well as to *provide flexible space that can be adapted over time.* Some ways to achieve flexibility are discussed in the next section.

## Planning Multiuse or Shared Facility Components

Planning multiuse or shared facility components enables a healthcare organization to use its space efficiently and to balance workload peaks and valleys. Examples of multiuse spaces include the following:

- *Acuity adaptable, or universal, patient rooms* can be adapted for most levels of acuity by altering staffing levels and equipment. This concept can reduce costly patient transfers during an increasingly short length of stay, provide improved continuity of care, and reduce medical errors.
- *Time-share clinic space* can be leased by physicians—for example, patient reception and intake areas, exam rooms, offices, and support space—by the day of week as needed, thus reducing fixed costs.
- *Multiuse procedure rooms* can accommodate various procedures as needed using different types of portable equipment, such as electrocardiogram (EKG) and ultrasound machines.
- *Redeploying space by shift* works in various ways, such as by using an adjacent occupational medicine clinic or same-day medical procedure unit for treating emergency department (ED) fast-track patients during the evening or night shift, or by holding ED patients in the surgery suite recovery area during the evening for observation or while waiting for an inpatient bed to become available.
- *Colocation of selected procedure rooms* allows rooms to share the same patient reception and intake, preparation, recovery, and support spaces—for example, the colocation of various imaging modalities, invasive cardiology and angiography, or endoscopy and surgery.

## Planning Flexible Space That Can Be Adapted over Time

Planning flexible space that can be adapted over time will accommodate shifts in program focus and fluctuating usage and can reduce long-term renovation costs. This type of planning includes space that can be easily adapted for a different functional use over time by replacing the equipment, adding a second bed, or reassigning offices and workstations to another department. In addition to acuity adaptable patient rooms, other examples of adaptable spaces include the following:

- *A flexible diagnostic and treatment center* has a central patient reception and intake area, preparation and recovery area, shared staff facilities, and a mix of large and small procedure rooms where equipment can be changed and upgraded over time. This innovation is in contrast to the traditional approach of planning dispersed and fragmented departments for radiology, computed tomography (CT), nuclear medicine, cardiology, and ultrasound.
- *Flexible customer service space* uses a one-stop shopping concept to accommodate admitting and registration, financial counseling, cashiering, scheduling, and other similar services that require face-to-face customer interaction. With flexible offices and cubicles (and cross-trained staff), services can be adapted to the customers' needs over time.
- *Generic administrative office suites* can be used by various administrative and support staff who do not require face-to-face customer contact. Space can be reassigned over time in response to organizational changes, thus eliminating department turf issues and improving overall space use.

## Unbundling Selected Services

Rather than embedding everything into the hospital structure, unbundling selected services can not only reduce an organization's initial capital investment but also facilitate future space reallocation, contraction, and expansion as workloads, staffing, and operational processes change over time. Some examples include the following:

- Relocation of routine, high-volume outpatient services in separate facilities (on or off campus) with dedicated parking and convenient access—for example, primary care clinics; selected high-volume outpatient services; or recurring or chronic outpatient services such as rehabilitation, chemotherapy, and dialysis
- Consolidation of building support services into a separate service building—for example, supply, processing, and distribution functions—using space that is less expensive to construct and renovate as operational systems, technology, and work processes change

◆ Relocation of administrative offices for staff who are not involved in direct patient care outside the hospital (on-site or off-site) in less expensive and adaptable office building space

## Leasing Space

Leasing space when appropriate, rather than buying or building, allows an organization to limit its capital investment and long-term risk. This strategy may include leasing space off-site for administrative offices and new or expanding outpatient programs. Some healthcare organizations may choose to lease space such as a hotel conference room or a school auditorium for periodic in-service or community education in lieu of constructing an education center on the hospital campus. Interior systems furniture and other building elements may also be leased by making an arrangement with a manufacturer to take stewardship over the product's life, including putting it together, refreshing it, and recycling it for a reasonable fee. Some healthcare organizations also keep up with changes in technology by leasing imaging equipment or by paying based on its use rather than buying the equipment outright.

## Building a Flexible Infrastructure

Using long-span joists and interstitial space (although not generally addressed in predesign planning) provides a cost-effective way to adapt to ongoing changes over the life of a building. When you embed everything in the building so that the pipes and wires are inside the walls, floors, and ceiling, reconfiguring any space without major construction is almost impossible. If you build your hospital more like a shopping center, with a huge superstructure and interiors that can come and go at will, you will have an adaptable tool for delivering healthcare.

# DEVELOPING SPACE STANDARDS AND PLANNING GENERIC SPACES

Future flexibility can also be achieved by developing generic space standards for rooms that accommodate similar functions. Cost savings will ultimately occur, as these rooms are similarly sized and finished instead of tailored to individual occupants, though the actual equipment may vary over time. Examples of generic spaces include the following:

- Private patient rooms (acuity adaptable)
- Small procedure rooms (ultrasound and EKG)
- Large imaging and procedure rooms (CT, positron emission tomography, and nuclear medicine)
- Interventional and surgical procedure rooms (cardiac catheterization, electrophysiology, angiography, peripheral vascular procedures, and invasive and minimally invasive surgery)
- Medical procedure cubicles (transfusions, chemotherapy, liver biopsies, recovery from conscious sedation, and fast-track emergency treatment)
- Administrative workstations, cubicles, private offices, and conference rooms

## REDESIGNING THE HEALTHCARE CAMPUS

A healthcare campus should be configured to reflect the needs of the community and allow the organization to compete in its market. Some large comprehensive campuses accommodate a variety of components of an integrated delivery system. These elements may include an acute care hospital; physician offices in one or more medical office buildings; a rehabilitation center; a skilled nursing facility; a wellness or complementary medicine center; and staff amenities such as a child day care center, a fitness center, and an education center. Other campuses focus exclusively on routine and acute ambulatory care and short-stay services.

Satellite ambulatory facilities, which have proliferated in recent years, are important for a variety of reasons. They help organizations tap unserved markets for primary care, they expand care in remote areas, and they provide growth opportunities for hospitals with limited expansion potential. Generally, outpatient workloads in satellite facilities should be large enough to justify redundant equipment and staff duplication—or they should earn enough incremental revenue to offset increased operational costs (Hayward 2015).

Healthcare campuses are being redesigned with a variety of distinct but connected functional components to facilitate short-term and long-range flexibility. When new construction is planned, these components are frequently unbundled to provide the least expensive and most appropriate construction for each function, depending on the requisite Life Safety Code compliance, corridor width, and infrastructure requirements. Potential buildings or facility components for the flexible healthcare campus include the following:

- Patient care units for overnight and multiple-day stays, day recovery centers, and shared diagnostic and treatment services (inpatient and outpatient) in a structure built to traditional hospital building codes
- One or more adjoining medical office buildings (built as outpatient facilities) for physician specialists and related outpatient services
- Specialty centers of excellence to provide one-stop shopping for targeted clinical services, such as cancer centers, heart centers, women's health centers, and sports medicine centers
- Separate facilities (on or off campus) with dedicated parking for primary care; routine outpatient diagnostic services; and chronic or recurring care such as outpatient physical therapy, dialysis, and behavioral health
- A separate service center for materials management functions that may be supported by an off-site warehouse, kitchen, medical device reprocessing center, and laundry facility
- An administrative office building for administrative and support staff who are not involved in direct patient care or face-to-face customer contact

Other freestanding components may include an education center, fitness center, and a day care facility for the children or elderly dependents of employees. Complementary medicine and retail services may also be provided, combined with or adjacent to high-volume traffic areas such as the hospital main entrance or a medical office building. Long-term care and assisted living facilities may even be provided as part of a very large "campus of care."

## REFERENCE

Hayward, C. 2015. *SpaceMed Guide: A Space Planning Guide for Healthcare Facilities*, 3rd ed. Ann Arbor, MI: HA Ventures.

# CHAPTER 16

# Ensuring Success: Optimizing
# Your Capital Investments

*Long-range planning does not deal with future decisions,*
*but with the future of present decisions.*

—Peter F. Drucker (1974)

WHETHER YOU ARE embarking on a major hospital replacement project, reconfiguring your current facilities, or simply upgrading a specific department or service line, the following summary guidelines should help you optimize your capital investments in facilities and increase your likelihood of success.

## DEPLOY A FORMAL PREDESIGN PLANNING PROCESS

The primary purpose of this book is to communicate the importance of the predesign planning process. Decisions made during this stage of facility planning have the greatest impact on long-term operational costs and future flexibility, in addition to the initial cost of the bricks and mortar. Whether you use a top-down or a bottom-up approach, integrating facility planning with your strategic (market) analysis, operations improvement, and technology planning efforts will allow you to make decisions with confidence and to move quickly into implementation.

## RETHINK CURRENT ORGANIZATIONAL AND OPERATIONAL MODELS AND USE OF TECHNOLOGY

The investment of significant dollars in new or renovated facilities is a rare opportunity for an organization to rethink its current patient care delivery model, operational systems and processes, and use of technology. Department managers should be encouraged to visualize delivering patient care beyond their individual silos. Cross-departmental task forces should be assembled to focus on common patient needs and operational processes to enhance customer satisfaction, provide efficient resource use, and promote future flexibility.

## SEPARATE PERCEPTION FROM REALITY

Because many factors affect patient and staff perception of inadequate facilities, understanding the actual facility issues before investing millions of dollars in renovation or new construction is important. A foundation of data and rigorous analyses should support the wish lists of department managers and physicians. At the same time, the relationship of the initial first impression to customer satisfaction should not be overemphasized.

## DEVELOP REALISTIC RETURN-ON-INVESTMENT ASSUMPTIONS

In the past, many healthcare organizations employed the "if you build it, they will come" approach to facility planning. Although some organizations were successful, others were faced with underused facilities and increased operational costs as revenues remained flat. An investment in healthcare facilities should be based on a sound business plan that forecasts future revenue and anticipates future operational costs.

## USE INDUSTRY BENCHMARKS, RULES OF THUMB, AND BEST PRACTICES FOR VALIDATION

The use of industry benchmarks and rules of thumb, along with a review of best practices around the country and internationally, provides external validation of your plans and may introduce your organization to new concepts and opportunities.

The use of industry benchmarks and rules of thumb is particularly important when you employ a bottom-up planning process or when department managers have a long tenure with a single organization. Alternately, when a top-down approach is used, the leadership's vision must be communicated to the staff, who will eventually occupy the new facilities. Site visits to other healthcare facilities and conversations with department managers and physicians who have implemented innovative operational concepts and technologies can save untold future operational and capital dollars.

## FOCUS ON THE CUSTOMER

Although providing superb patient care is always the focus of a healthcare organization's mission, patients are not the only customers. Physicians, employees, payers, and family members and visitors all have unique needs that must be considered during the facility planning process.

## OPTIMIZE CURRENT AND FUTURE FLEXIBILITY

As described in chapter 11, there are a number of ways to optimize current and future flexibility that can reduce short-term capital and operational costs and minimize long-term renovation costs.

## REFERENCE

Drucker, P. F. 1974. *Management: Tasks, Responsibilities, Practices.* New York: Harper & Row.

# Index

Note: Italicized page locators refer to exhibits.

Furniture: leasing, 184
Future capacity: rationale for potential projects and, 108
Future demand forecasts: capacity assessment linked to, 47–48
Future facility configuration drawings, 105, *106*

Generic spaces: planning, 184–85
Gift shops, 55
Gross space: net space *vs.,* 25, *26,* 27–28, 136
*Guidelines for Design and Construction of Hospitals and Outpatient Facilities* (FGI *Guidelines*), 130

Handicap accessibility standards, state and local, 130
Health agency codes: state, 130
Healthcare campus. *See* Campus planning
Healthcare executives: predesign planning and, 11
Healthcare reform: consolidation and, 7; new planning environment and, 2–3
*Healthcare Strategic Planning* (Zuckerman), 37
Healthcare systems: consolidation of, 7
Health informatics, 5
Health Insurance Portability and Accountability Act (HIPAA), 4
Health safety: rationale for potential projects and, 107
High bed need scenarios, 39–40, *41, 43*
HIPAA. *See* Health Insurance Portability and Accountability Act
Home base: providing, for families and visitors, 102
Home health agencies: proliferation of, 4
Hospital-centric model: population-centric model *vs.,* 4, 40
Hospital licensing rules, state, 130
Hospitals: closures of, 40, 87; consolidations of, 40; downsizings of hospital-based departments and, 40, 96; facility planning issues for services or departments in, 83–84; flexible infrastructure for, 184; future bed need scenarios comparison, *41;* inpatient care space in, 95; occupancy rates in, 40; optimizing reimbursement for, 7; reconfiguring diagnostic services in, 57–58;

replacement, planning from the ground up, 115; traditional facility planning process and, 2. *See also* Acute care hospitals; Community hospitals; Case study: consolidating two acute care hospitals; Multihospital systems
Hotel services (or building support services), 63
Hub-and-spoke model: customer service center and, 102; hotel reception–desk concept, 23, 57
Human resources departments: reengineering of operations and, 6
Hybrid operating room, 59

Imaging equipment: leasing, 184
Imaging procedure space: integrating with surgical procedure space, 59
Imaging services: location for, 58
Imaging studies, 5
Implementation planning: strategic planning and, 37
Inadequate facilities: perception of, 99, *100*
Incremental approach, 70
Inflation factor: adding to base construction cost, 113
Information technology (IT): advances in, 5, 51–52; integrating facility planning with investments in, 49. *See also* Electronic health records; Internet
Infrastructure: flexible, 184; major issues for, 35, 36; strategic planning for, 38; upgrading, 94, 97
Inpatient beds: declining demand for, 4
Inpatient care: fragmentation of, 95
Inpatient floor: typical layout of, 21
Inpatient nursing units, 18, 36, 84; data collection for, 28–29; department gross square feet of, 34; design capacity of, 29; inventory and analysis of, 73, *75;* programming, 133–34, *135*
Inpatient rooms: building codes and, 130
Inpatients: outpatients *vs.,* 97
Inpatient space: redeploying or downgrading, 22
Inpatient transfers: minimizing, 82
Institute of Medicine (IOM): *To Err Is Human* report, 7–8
Institution-wide operations improvement initiatives, 49–50

Multihospital systems, 64; eliminating surplus capacity in, 87; political, emotional, and regulatory issues related to, 90

Multihospital system ten-year capital investment strategy (case study), 139–50; current bed complement, *145*; detailed project phasing and implementation plan, 150; existing hospital sites and characteristics, *141*; facility planning process, 142; key facility priorities, 143, 145–46; long-range facility development scenarios, 146–47; major facility assets and liabilities by campus, 142–43, *144*; market dynamics and future bed need, 143; ten-year capital investment strategy, 147, *148, 149*; three acute care campuses, description of, 139–40; 2015 capital investment strategy, 140, 142

Multiple-bed rooms or wards, 42

Multispecialty group practices, 7

Multiuse facility components: planning, 182

Needs assessment: eliminating surplus capacity, 87–91; evaluating facility capacity, 71, 73–74, 76, 78–79; key facility issues and priorities, 83–85; key questions to ask in, 67; matrices used in, 85, *86*; outpatient population and, 79–80; summarizing space requirements, 83; tools and techniques in, 68–71; understanding the space planning process, 67–68

Neonatal intensive care units (NICUs), 70; modeling space for different sizes and configurations of, *72*

Net assignable (or usable) area, 28

Net space: gross space *vs.*, 25, *26*, 27–28, 136

Net square feet (NSF), 25, *26*, 27, 28, 68; ambulatory care facility planning case study, 152, *154*; emergency expansion evaluation, 158

Net-to-department gross space conversion factor, 27

New consumerism, 8–9

New facility: planning, from the ground up, 115

New planning environment, 2–9; aging facilities and, 8; consolidation in, 7; convergence of diagnostic, interventional imaging, and surgical procedures in, 5–6; electronic health records in, 4–5; fluctuating demand/utilization and, 3–4; healthcare reform and, 2–3; information technology advances and, 5; media attention to patient safety and, 7–8; new consumerism and, 8–9; operations reengineering, process improvement, and, 6–7; reimbursement and, 7; turf wars and, 6

*Non-Architect's Guide to Major Capital Projects: Planning, Designing, and Delivering New Buildings* (Waite), 16

NSF. *See* Net square feet

Nursing units: capacity analysis, example of, *75*; reconfiguration of, 94, 95–96; size of, 21

Observation beds: same-day-stay patients and, 42, 44

Observation units: developing, 60–61

Occupancy planning, 134

Open-bay designs, 70–71

Operating rooms: hybrid, 59

Operational and space programming, 9, *9*

Operational configuration models: new, 53

Operational costs: predesign planning and impact on, *12*

Operational efficiency: rationale for potential projects and, 108

Operational processes: facility planning and, 84

Operational programs/programming: components of, 118; defining, 117–18; detailed, preparing, 117; for endoscopy suite, example, 118–25; inpatient nursing units, 133–34, *135*; relationship of, to subsequent documentation, 134; supplementary conceptual diagrams and, 130–31, *131*; ten common pitfalls in, 134, 136–37

Operational space programming: bottom-up approach to, 131, *132,* 132–33; top-down approach to, 131, *132,* 133

Operations improvement, 9, *9*

Operations reengineering: consolidation of traditional hospital departments through, 49–50

Organizational charts: flatter, 6

Organizational direction: strategic planning and, 37

Strategy formulation: strategic planning and, 37

Surgeons: workload projections and, 45

Surgery: forecasting workload for, 45, *46*

Surgical procedures: convergence of diagnostic and interventional imaging with, 5–6; integrating imaging procedure space with space for, 59

Surplus capacity: consolidating physician practices, 88; eliminating, issues associated with, 87–91; eliminating empty beds, 87–88; integrating and restructuring clinical services, 88; major consolidation issues separated from nonissues, 89–90; overview of, 87; political, emotional, and regulatory issues tied to, 90–91; reducing building support space, 89; for space and equipment, 38

Surveys, 69

Technology: common institution-wide systems and, 50–51; facility planning and, 84; investing in, 9, *9*; mobile, 5, 52; outdated, 84–85; rethinking use of, 188; telecommunications, 52; wireless, 5. *See also* Electronic health records; Information technology; Internet

Telemedicine, 5, 52

Telepresence: eICU and, 61

Time-share clinic space, 182

*To Err Is Human* (Institute of Medicine), 7–8

Top-down approach: leadership's vision and, 189; to operational space programming, 131, *132*, 133

Total project cost, 112–13

Traditional facility planning process: problems with, 1–2

Traffic flow, 18

Treatment spaces: characteristics of, 22; major, 33

Turf wars: new planning environment and, 6

Underground utilities, 17

Uninsured population: Affordable Care Act and, 4

Unpredictable healthcare environment: flexibility and, 181

Usable square feet, 28

Utilization: facility planning and analysis of, 38–39; fluctuating, new planning environment and, 3–4

Vacant spaces, 38

Valet parking, 64

Validation of plans: industry benchmarks, rules of thumb, and best practices for, 188–89

Vascular surgeons, 6

Videoconferencing, 25

Virtual workplaces, 52

Visitors: circulation system and, 18; signage and, 102

Voice communication, 5, 52

Waite, Phillip S., 11, 16

Wayfinding, 17, 51, 64, 65; customer service center and, 54; improving, 101–2. *See also* Signage

Wireless technologies, 5

Workload: capacity, facility planning and, 83; composition, space program and, 129; projections of, 45, *46*

Young consumers, 8–9

Zero-based budget approach, 70

Zuckerman, Alan M., 37

# About the Author

Cynthia Hayward, AIA, is principal and founder of Hayward & Associates LLC in Ann Arbor, Michigan, a national consulting firm specializing in predesign planning for healthcare facilities. She has assisted hundreds of diverse healthcare organizations over the past 30 years in planning their capital investments economically and efficiently. For 20 years, she was a partner with a healthcare management consulting firm (Chi Systems, Inc., which became The Chi Group) until she founded Hayward & Associates. Her unique approach integrates facility planning with market demand and clinical service planning, operations improvement, and investments in new equipment and information technology.

In addition to her consulting activities, Ms. Hayward has a long history in research and development relative to healthcare facility planning. In the mid-1970s, she was part of a team contracted by the US Department of Health and Human Services to develop a generic healthcare facility planning process for hospitals across the United States. In the early 1980s, she served as project director for a five-year contract with National Health and Welfare Canada to develop a series of space planning methodologies for healthcare facilities—the Evaluation and Space Programming Methodology Series—that were used throughout North America over the subsequent decade. Ms. Hayward is also the author of the *SpaceMed Guide: A Space Planning Guide for Healthcare Facilities* (see www.spacemed.com), which includes a step-by-step workbook and a CD-ROM with detailed space planning templates.

She has been a speaker at regional, national, and international conferences on issues relating to predesign planning and capital investment, including conferences sponsored by the American College of Healthcare Executives, the Healthcare Financial Management Association, the American Hospital Association, and the American Institute of Architects.

Ms. Hayward has a master of architecture degree from the University of Michigan and is a licensed architect (Michigan). She is also a member of the American Institute of Architects and a founding member of the American College of Healthcare Architects.